AF335726

MEDICAL LICENSING IN AMERICA, 1650–1965

MEDICAL LICENSING IN AMERICA, 1650-1965

by Richard Harrison Shryock

The Johns Hopkins Press, Baltimore, Maryland

*In memory of my respected
colleagues, Alexandre Koyré of Paris,
and Juan B. Lastres of Lima*

PREFACE 🙠

In 1649 the Province of Massachusetts, barely twenty years after its original settlement, adopted a law to regulate the activities of "Chirurgeons, Midwives, Physitians or others" who were "imployed at any time about the bodye of men, women or children, for preservation of life, or health." No such persons were to practice "without the advice and consent of such as are skillful in the same Art (if such may be had) or at least some of the wisest and gravest then present"; and if these rules were not observed, violators were subjected to "such severe punishment as the nature of the fact may deserve." This Act, as vague as it was well-intentioned, soon proved ineffective; for within four years a petition was presented to the General Court (Assembly), noting that the unskilled continued to practice "to the detriment of many." The petitioner therefore urged the court to restrain such persons until they could be approved by "authorized Physitians and Chirurgeons," after which they should be licensed by magistrates "to practice the time they are resident here" [Boston]. Those who ignored such regulation could be fined by the court.[1]

There is no evidence that this petition was embodied in law or that, in any case, acts of this nature were enforced during the ensuing century—either in Massachusetts or in any of the other English colonies. Yet one finds in these statements anticipation of difficulties which were to confront American medicine for the next three centuries, and doubtless will continue to do so in the future. The problem involved was that of protecting both the public and the profession through medical education and licensure. To be more specific, how could American society reconcile within this area—one is tempted to say within this arena—the sometimes conflicting interests

---

[1] F. R. Packard, *History of Medicine in the United States* (reprint, 1931 ed.; New York: Hafner, 1963), I, 166 f.

of professional leaders on the one hand and of lay spokesmen on the other?

Several other aspects of the public relations of medicine, notably medical costs and medical ethics, have been equally vital and equally troublesome. There were to be times, indeed, when one of these issues would take precedence over the other. It is not surprising, for example, that colonial laws and court actions were more often concerned with fees than with the quality of services.[2] Differences in the number of laws, however, do not necessarily indicate the relative significance of such matters.

This study focuses on the dual theme of education and licensure—using each of those terms in a broad sense. It relates primarily to the American scene, although European institutions must be noted either as models or as points of departure for developments in this country. Isolated entirely from this background the transatlantic story would be superficial, if not actually inexplicable.

As those writing on the professions point out, occupational groups have exhibited common forms of behavior when they arrived at similar levels of development. Thus, a vocation which evolved specialized skills and aspired to higher status would seek to limit membership to those who attained such skills and employed them in an ethical manner. Organization was at first informal, but as soon as conditions permitted, members demanded testing of those admitted to what in time became formal bodies.[3]

[2] *Ibid.*, chap. 3; W. B. Blanton, *Medicine in Virginia in the Seventeenth Century* (Richmond: William Byrd Press, 1930), chap. 12.

[3] See A. M. Carr-Saunders and P. A. Wilson, *The Professions* [history of, in England] (London: Oxford Univ. Press, 1933), *passim;* G. G. Reader and Mary E. W. Gross, "The Sociology of Medicine," pp. 242–46, and E. C. Hughes, "The Study of Occupations," pp. 447–52, in R. K. Merton, L. Groom, and L. S. Cottrell, Jr., eds., *Sociology Today* (New York: Basic Books, 1959); and B. Barber, "Some Problems in the Sociology of the Professions," *Daedalus* (Fall, 1963), pp. 671–73. Concise but stimulating is R. Merton's *Some Thoughts on Professions in American Society* (Providence: Brown Univ. Studies, XXXVII, 1960).

An apparent exception in the United States was made in the case of college and university professors, who were rarely if ever licensed. This was an ill-defined group. Was a professor of chemistry, for example, a chemist or a teacher? Or was a medical professor primarily a physician or an academician? Answers were apt to depend on time and place. True, certain degrees were finally required of nearly all professors in strong institutions. And in this respect, the accrediting of professors is now controlled by universities; much as was that of physicians by medical schools during the greater part of the last century.

For the present purpose, the best illustrations of historic guilds—in a broad sense of that term—are provided by the traditional "learned professions." A comparative study of licensure in law, in medicine, and in divinity might prove enlightening, though in some respects the first two of these offer the more meaningful contrasts. One assumes, therefore, that some promise inheres in a comparative history of the legal and medical professions, and pertinent articles have been published in this connection.[4] Better studies have now appeared on the history of law and of the native "bench and bar," and from these the medical observer may draw his own conclusions.[5] Meantime, despite statements that "practically nothing is known about the history of the professions in the United States,"[6] considerable literature on the medical theme has appeared over the past century, and particularly during recent decades. Hence, material needed for comparative studies is available.[7]

[4] E.g., A. Z. Reed, "Restrictions upon Professions Prior to the Civil War," *The Bar Examiner,* II (1933), 31–32; and, more recently, the significant studies listed in *Law and Society* (supplement to summer issue of *Social Problems;* Boston: 1965), pp. 6, 10, and 57.

[5] E.g., R. B. Morris, *Studies in the History of American Law* (2d ed.; Philadelphia: J. M. Mitchell Co., 1959); A. H. Chroust, *The Rise of the Legal Profession in America,* 2 vols. (Norman: Univ. of Oklahoma Press, 1965).

[6] Oscar Handlin, Foreword to D. H. Calhoun, *Professional Lives in America* . . . (Cambridge: Harvard Univ. Press, 1965).

[7] See, e.g., "Professional History," in Genevieve Miller, ed., *Bibliography of the History of Medicine of the United States and Canada, 1939–1960* (Baltimore:

Comparisons of law and medicine exhibit two tendencies which could have been anticipated. When marked changes occurred, internal to one guild as such, analogous trends rarely appeared within the other. But when a profession was influenced by its social environment, the other guild—operating within the same setting—usually was similarly influenced. Occasional comments will be made on such instances although no systematic comparisons can be attempted.

Finally, such terms as "medicine" or "practitioner," as used here, do not cover several fields which logically might have been included. Thus, dentistry, pharmacy, and veterinary medicine are excluded, partly because these evolved as distinct professions and partly because, in any case, there is no end to the complexities of even a limited exposition.

I have been indebted, in preparing this study, to Dr. Katharine R. Sturgis and to Dr. Owsei Temkin for helpful suggestions; to Dr. John P. Hubbard for providing materials on the National Board of Medical Examiners; and to Dr. Whitfield J. Bell, Jr. and Dr. Marion Elderton for locating valuable sources. Mrs. Julianne Pearson prepared the typescript.

RICHARD HARRISON SHRYOCK

Philadelphia
November, 1966

The Johns Hopkins Press, 1964) pp. 343–49; also other sections in this volume covering only two recent decades. On the extensive earlier literature on medical licensure in the United States, as well as abroad, see *Index Catalogue of the Library of the Surgeon General* (Washington: U.S. Army, Gov't Printing Office, 1887), VIII, 951–55; second ser. (1905), X, 469–85.

CONTENTS &

MEDICAL LICENSING IN AMERICA,
1650—1965

CHAPTER I „ EARLY LICENSING AND SUBSEQUENT DECADENCE: 1650–1875

Except for small facilities maintained by individuals, there were no medical institutions in this country for nearly 150 years after the first settlements appeared. In contrast, courts were soon set up to enforce the law, although legal training was suspect and untrained judges depended more on common sense than on common law. In this respect, the legal and medical situations were similar, reflecting the limitations of plain people who found themselves temporarily beyond the reach of English facilities and regulations. In new communities there was often a lack of men with any pretence to medical education, and those who just undertook practice were welcomed if they inspired confidence. Women as well as men served as general practitioners among their neighbors. And in the southern colonies, plantation mistresses, overseers, and an occasional slave—perhaps with "a gift from the Lord"—practiced without pay.

In the case of medicine, even the best of so-called doctors were usually trained only by apprenticeship. This procedure probably became more common after 1700, and in the process women seem to have dropped out of the picture except as midwives. According to later tradition, most apprenticed men became sound practitioners—fortunately ignorant of theories but blessed by good sense and experience. Americans, it is still said, are a practical folk and this made their "doctors" at least as effective as were formally trained Europeans.[8] If this

[8] So said Nathaniel Chapman, first president of the American Medical Association (AMA), in 1820 (*Phila. Jour. Med. and Phys. Sciences,* I [1820], 9); Oliver Wendell Holmes in the 1860s (*Currents and Cross-Currents in Medical Science* [Boston: 1861] pp. 5–8); F. H. Garrison in the 1920s (*History of Medicine* [4th ed.; Philadelphia: 1929], pp. 303 ff.); Henry E. Sigerist expressed a somewhat similar view in the 1930s (*American Medicine* [New York: Norton, 1934], p. 41); and Daniel J. Boorstin in the 1950s (*The Americans: The Colonial Experience* [New York: Random House, 1958], pp. 233 ff.).

view is sound, one wonders why, well before 1800, so many medical leaders urged that educational and licensing requirements should be introduced on this side of the Atlantic?

Actually, of course, the evidence is conflicting. Many laymen thought well of their medical advisers but the question remains: Were they good judges of professional merit? It seems more likely that the few physicians who secured degrees abroad, and so knew both the American and European scenes, were better qualified to attempt appraisals. Such testimony was more than critical: it was damning. "Frequently," declared Dr. William Douglass of Boston, in 1753, "there is *more Danger* from the Physician than from the Distemper."[9] And Dr. John Morgan in founding the first native medical school twelve years later, said that even in large towns many practitioners were " in a pitiful state of ignorance." He was alarmed by the havoc wrought by these men and appealed to them to withhold their "exterminating hands."[10] Some fifty years after that, Dr. John Stearns, president of the New York State Medical Society, declared in retrospect that: "With a few, honorable exceptions . . . the practitioners were ignorant, degraded and contemptible"—strong language even for that era.[11]

Although disdain may be partly ascribed to the pride of holders of a degree, practitioners lacking formal training were likewise critical at times. A group in Connecticut, to be mentioned below, referred in 1780 to "that unhappy Slaughter which is daily made amongst our fellow citizens by the barbarous hands of medicasters." And even laymen were some-

[9] *A Summary of . . . the Present State of the British Settlements in North-America* (Boston: 1753), II, 351. See also Blanton, *Medicine in Virginia* (n. 2, above). pp. 97 f.

[10] *A Discourse upon the Institution of Medical Schools in America* (Philadelphia: 1765; reprinted Baltimore: The Johns Hopkins Press, 1937), pp. 23–27. Jefferson's low opinion of doctors, as well as of medicine, is also well known; see, e.g., his *Notes on Virginia,* W. Peden, ed. (Chapel Hill: Univ. of N.C. Press, 1955), pp. 285 f.

[11] Presidential Address, New York State Medical Society *Trans.,* I (1818) 139.

times caustic. In a passage often quoted, the historian William Smith stated in 1757 that: "Few physicians among us are eminent for their skill. Quacks abound like locusts in Egypt. . . . This," he added, "is less to be wondered at as the profession is under no kind of Regulation. Any man at his pleasure sets up for Physician, Apothecary, and Chirurgen."[12]

Clearly, Smith was aware that there was such a thing as "regulation" in the Old World and implied that it should be introduced into the colonies. Now that colonial towns were as large as English provincial cities—yet far more distant from London— he and others wished to import "medical police" into the colonial provinces. The first efforts to do this involved an adjustment of British practice to American circumstances. Later, institutions in both countries continued to change, sometimes diverging but often arriving finally at similar destinations.

In western Europe the three groups mentioned by William Smith had emerged gradually from medieval backgrounds and had long since coalesced into formal bodies. Strictly speaking, the organizations of apothecaries and surgeons had remained guilds in the medieval sense, while physicians had become members of a learned profession. London physicians, trained at the universities, ministered to the upper classes and enjoyed a status superior to that of apothecaries who kept drug shops and of surgeons who worked with their hands. But in small towns and rural areas, such specialization was rarely feasible, and by the eighteenth century—if not before—all three groups tended to pursue general practice.[13]

[12] *History of the Province of New York* . . . (London: 1757), p. 212. Morris, *History of American Law* (n. 5, above), notes similar popular ridicule of lawyers. On the Connecticut practitioners, see n. 35, below.

[13] R. S. Roberts, "The Personnel and Practice of Medicine in Tudor and Stuart England: Pt. I, The Provinces," *Medical History*, VI, no. 4 (October, 1962), 363–82. On the medieval origins of medical guilds, see V. L. Bulloch, *The Development of Medicine as a Profession* . . . (New York: Hafner, 1966), chap. 4.

Physicians were accorded the greatest prestige, probably not so much in relation to technical knowledge as in recognition of social and cultural advantages. Yet it may have been because of the common type of service in most areas that many practitioners were called "doctors" whether or not they held degrees.[14] Thus, in medicine (as, at times, in law), the term acquired a broader connotation than its strictly academic meaning; that is, it also was used to designate anyone who provided medical services. Even practitioners not addressed by this title in Britain, notably surgeons but also apothecaries, still might be referred to in the third person as doctors—a usage recalled in Wilkie Collins' *Moonstone* with its occasional references to "Mr. Candy, our doctor."

Italian ideas about state examinations and licensure had reached northern Europe toward the end of the Middle Ages, and all three medical groups sought official authority to carry out these procedures for their respective personnel. Actually, guilds had long exercised controls over their own membership, but this self-regulation came ultimately to be sanctioned by Church and State. The first national medical program in England was set up in 1510, when Parliament placed control in the hands of the Church. More precisely, bishops were authorized to examine and license physicians and surgeons throughout the realm. Those who were graduates of Oxford and Cambridge, however, could practice without episcopal approval, since learned professions had long been licensed by university faculties.[15] This privilege for holders of a degree persisted in England and appeared later within a different setting in the United States.

[14] Roberts (M. 13, above), p. 376.
[15] H. E. Sigerist, "The History of Medical Licensure," *Jour. Amer. Med. Assoc.*, vol. 104 (March 30, 1935); reprinted in M. I. Roemer, ed., *Henry E. Sigerist on the Sociology of Medicine* (New York: M.D. Publications, 1960), pp. 308–318.

Ecclesiastical control of medical licensure, which now seems strange, was logical enough at the time. Until the Renaissance outstanding physicians had usually been clergymen; moreover, episcopal authority extended throughout the kingdom and so provided, in principle, a national system. As a matter of fact, clergymen continued to practice or to publish medical works as late as the eighteenth century in both England and its colonies. As long as there were no widely enforced regulations, ordination—especially in a state church—conferred in effect a vague license to practice. At the least, it made such practice respectable in small communities. Recall, for example, the Reverend John Wesley in England and the Reverend Cotton Mather in New England.

Even before the law of 1510 was enacted, however, laymen were already taking over and the clerical role was thereafter a declining one. As early as 1518, the Crown turned to self-regulation by lay physicians in founding the Royal College of Physicians and giving it examining and licensing powers in or near the capital. These rights were extended in 1522 to cover all England. Similar authority over their respective groups was later granted to the London Company of Barber-Surgeons (1540) and the Surgeons' Company (1745), as well as to the London Society of Apothecaries founded in 1617; though it is not clear how effective any of these bodies were outside the London area. British laws, moreover, rarely forbade untrained persons from practicing; usually, only misrepresentation of status was penalized. The control of approved practice in the British Isles was thus left by Parliament to voluntary professional bodies. These included the old corporations of each medical guild in England, in Scotland, and in Ireland, and also the universities. Even a vestige of ecclesiastical tradition survived in licenses granted by the Archbishop of Canterbury.[16]

[16] Clear, summarized accounts of licensing within Britain will be found in F. N. L. Poynter and K. D. Keele, *A Short History of Medicine* (London: 1961),

Noteworthy, however, is the fact that neither Crown nor Parliament extended professional regulations to overseas provinces. At first, no doubt, most settlements were too small and scattered to justify efforts of this sort, but the situation had certainly changed by 1720 and there must have been other explanations. Political attitudes may have been responsible: imperial control over the colonies was lax during long periods. (In contrast, attempts were made to extend the medical code of Castile to the Spanish American colonies as early as the sixteenth century.) British policy and colonial attitudes, whatever their origins, had important consequences: each province was placed on its own in matters relating to medical practice. This fact had basic implications for later developments in the United States, but before discussing these outcomes, one must recall the later history of the medical guilds: how these fared at first in America and how they subsequently were transformed in both the Old World and the New.

It is often assumed that English distinctions broke down or were rejected in America, where conditions required each practitioner to serve as druggist and surgeon as well as internist. But one may ascribe the outcome simply to the fact that similar environments encouraged similar behavior on both sides of the Atlantic. The training and practice of "doctors" in rural America was similar in many ways to that of the village surgeons or apothecaries who took care of most Englishmen.[17] The

---

pp. 140 f.; and in Poynter, "The Influence of Government Legislation on Medical Practice in Britain," in the volume edited by him, *The Evolution of Medical Practice in Britain* (London: Pitman, 1961), pp. 5–15. See also Charles Newman, *The Evolution of Medical Education in the Nineteenth Century* (London: Oxford Univ. Press, 1957), pp. 4–25; and B. Spector, "The Growth of Medicine and the Letter of the Law," *Bull. of the Hist. of Med.,* vol. 26 (November, 1952), pp. 499–525.

[17] An Englishman visiting the United States in 1797 referred to "a man of good education [who] practices physic here, somewhat as our country apothecaries in England do, for which he is dubbed Doctor." Sir William Craigie and J. R. Hulbert, eds., *A Dictionary of American English* (Chicago: 1940), II, 786. The English "country apothecaries," were condemned as severely as were American "docs"; see John Chapman, *Medical Institutions of the United Kingdom* (London: 1870), p. 34.

chief difference was that physicians proper—as known in London—rarely appeared in the colonies for more than a century. Physicians, like the upper classes in general, did not migrate overseas, and for a long period no American towns were large enough to train such men on their own behalf.

In consequence, with nearly all Americans practicing like British surgeon-apothecaries, there was little need to use guild titles. In formal language, distinctions between "physic" and "surgery" survived, and some men were simply called "surgeons" or "barber-surgeons." But in ordinary usage the terms "doctor," "surgeon," and "physician" came to be employed almost interchangeably. Americans, unlike the British, even addressed all such men as "doctor," with a sort of equalitarian abandon.[18] In the meantime, the word "apothecary" preserved or reverted to its original meaning and was gradually given up by general practitioners. When a few colonists returned home with European degrees, after 1740, their status was analogous to that of English physicians located in the provinces and they behaved accordingly; that is, they enjoyed prestige but practiced much as did all other "doctors."

Colonists abroad observed that Scottish medical faculties, following the Continental tradition, were located in universities and granted M.B. (bachelor of medicine) or M.D. degrees. But Americans who sought training in Edinburgh, because of its facilities and faculty, noted quite a different situation in England, where the universities ignored modern science in general and medical advances in particular. They failed to provide clinical teaching during the later eighteenth century; hence strictly medical education was obtainable only in the London hospitals. Schools formed within several of these small institu-

[18] Craigie, *A Dictionary of American English* (n. 17, above), p. 786. For similar usage as early as 1721, see R. H. Fitz, "Zabdiel Boylston, Inoculator," *Bull. of the Johns Hopkins Hosp.* XXII (1911), 13. British scorn for the American use of the word "doctor" continued into the next century, see e.g. R. K. Webb, *Harriet Martineau* . . . (New York: Columbia Univ. Press, 1960), p. 136.

tions, offering clinical and surgical training but lacking university connections and degree-granting privileges. Not until well into the nineteenth century were these desiderata offered through the newly formed University of London.[19]

Students from all parts of the United Kingdom resorted to the London hospital-schools or to supplementary "private" schools, maintained by members of the clinical staffs. Among them were "Oxbridge" graduates who were licensed by the universities and might be elected fellows of the Royal College. Since the latter was an examining body, it licensed those who passed its tests, and thus many men trained only in hospital-schools became licentiates. Such men claimed a right to election as fellows, and although few attained this status they brought democratic pressures to bear on the college. Meantime, men who had a more limited education and took the less rigorous examinations of the Society of Apothecaries were licensed by that guild. In this way, future physicians and apothecaries—and surgeons for that matter—came to study within the same hospital environment. As early as the 1790s efforts were made to reform medical practice by up-grading the apothecaries and surgeons—those who actually served the majority of the people. The Apothecaries' Act of 1815 is usually said to have authorized general practice by that group, even in London, though this law has recently been viewed as a reactionary measure which still kept apothecaries subordinate to physicians.[20]

What happened thereafter, in any case, was that guild lines became blurred and were replaced by distinctions between

[19] Newman, *Evolution of Medical Education* (n. 16, above), pp. 112–16.

[20] On guild distinctions and types of schools in London, see Bernice Hamilton, "The Medical Professions in the Eighteenth Century," *The Economic Hist. Rev.*, second ser., IV (1951), 141–69; and L. S. King, *The Medical World of the Eighteenth Century* (Chicago: Univ. of Chicago Press, 1958), chap. 1. On the hospital and private schools, see also Carr-Saunders, *The Professions* (n. 3, above), p. 80. Medical reform, 1793–1815, is discussed in S. W. F. Holloway, "The Apothecaries' Act of 1815: A Reinterpretation—Pt. I, The Origins . . .," *Medical Hist.*, X (April, 1966), 107–29.

superior and ordinary grades within one profession. This trend
may be explained in part by the circumstances just mentioned:
namely, the common training experience in hospital-schools.
(Such institutions were founded in provincial cities as well as
in the metropolis after 1825.) Current scientific advances almost forced such training on practitioners, no matter what their
educational backgrounds. As noted, the older guild divisions
had been partly social and cultural in nature and these distinctions became less significant just to the extent that technical
knowledge became essential.

One may surmise that the merger of guilds was further encouraged by the growth of equalitarianism. If so, the trans-
formation involved occurred slowly and was never complete.
Upper-class patients in both the United Kingdom and the
United States still prefer upper-class physicians, and vice versa,[21]
but a partial shift in attitudes may have had some bearing on
the decline in formal distinctions. The outcome of all these
influences, converging on Britain after 1820, was that physicians
became in effect first-class, and apothecaries second-class practitioners.

The same distinctions within a single profession also took
form in continental Europe. In France, notably, the Revolution
of the 1790s swept away old medical faculties and corporations,
and the national government, which had already taken over
many hospitals from the Church, proceeded to set up state
medical schools. (This emphasis upon centralized control char-
acterized later Continental programs, in contrast to the Anglo-
Saxon bent for voluntary self-regulation.) Not surprisingly,
in France examinations and licensing also became functions of
national agencies. Provisions were made for both physicians,

---

[21] O. Simmons, *Social Status and Public Health* (New York: Social Sci. Res.
Council, 1958), p. 17. A brief, useful discussion of the transition to equalitarianism is given in B. Barber, "Change and the Social Stratification System in
Russia, Great Britain, and the United States," in B. Barber and Elinor Barber,
eds., *European Social Class* . . . (New York: Macmillan, 1965), pp. 137–45.

as first-class practitioners, and for *officiers de santé* who—taking briefer training and less severe examinations—were clearly a second-class group.[22] The latter type had its counterparts in other countries as well, as in the German *sekundär Arzte,* in the Russian *feldshers,* and in the British practitioners mentioned.

During the early nineteenth century, the upper-classes still assumed that second-class practice was good enough for the masses, while the masses may have thought it good enough for anyone—a plausible view as long as the resources of even the best men were so limited. By mid-century, however, scientific advances foreshadowed the more effective therapy to come, and middle-class humanitarianism encouraged more concern for the welfare of the poor. The outcome, eventually, was a conviction among reformers that every class should have access to the best in medicine. In these terms, all practitioners should be trained as well as possible and examined with equal care; ergo, admittedly second-grade "doctors" should be eliminated.

Just how the masses could afford the services of first-class physicians was not fully thought out in advance. Actually, compulsory health insurance was an eighteenth-century idea, formulated when the services of lower-grade practitioners were still taken for granted. But the idea was not widely applied before the 1880s. Conceivably, a decline in the number of second-class "doctors" was eventually a factor in the adoption of national insurance in Germany at that time. Higher licensing standards may have increased the cost of services, and by the same token the need for government aid in meeting these costs. Later, in other countries—as originally in Germany—

<hr>

[22] E. H. Ackerknecht, "Medical Education in 19th Century France," *Jour. of Med. Educ.,* vol. 32 (1957), pp. 148 ff.; see also Hardwick, *Medical Education and Practice* (n. 57, below), pp. 76–78, *passim,* for the French program by 1880, as well as those in other European countries.

medical reform was usually a precursor to medical care programs.[23]

To be more specific, it was Germany a generation before the 1880s—which took the lead in eliminating second-class training programs. Despite disillusionment among liberals during the Revolution of 1848, Prussia began to require uniform educational standards in 1852 and its example was soon followed by other German principalities. Each *Land* maintained its own universities, and under new laws required the same state examinations and licenses for all physicians.[24] Appeals for medical reform were also voiced, at the time, in the United Kingdom and in the United States; but effective response was delayed in both of these countries—apparently, in part, because of the Anglo-Saxon preference for voluntary regulation.

It is when one turns from general trends to particular aspects of education and licensure, that phenomena peculiar to the United States become apparent. Under the British Empire, as noted, each colony had been autonomous in medical affairs and acted accordingly. The first attempts to organize American practitioners had preceded efforts to found medical schools. Short-lived, local societies, open to more or less respectable "doctors," had appeared in various towns between the 1730s and 1760s, just as the early bar associations were formed by prominent lawyers in Boston and New York during the 1740s.[25] About mid-century, after London-trained lawyers returned to the colonies, these bodies even began to set educa-

[23] See articles by George Rosen, notably "Hospitals, Medical Care, and Social Policy during the French Revolution," *Bull. of the Hist. of Med.*, XXX (1956), 139; for the long perspective, R. H. Shryock, "Medicine and Society in the Nineteenth Century," *Jour. of World Hist.*, V (1959), 122 ff., reprinted in G. S. Metraux and F. Crovzet, eds., *The Nineteenth Century World* . . . (New York: New Amer. Libr., 1963), pp. 193–253.

[24] Paul Diepgen, *Geschichte der Medizin*, (Berlin: De Gruyter, 1959), II, 70. For the German background, see, e.g., C. L. P. Trüb, "Die Geschichtliche Entwicklung des ärztlichen Standeswesens in Deutschland" (1823–1932), *Medizinische Monatschrift*, Jahrgang 15, Heft 7 (July, 1961), pp. 478 ff.

[25] Chroust, *Legal Profession in America* (n. 5, above), pp. 130–35.

tional requirements and to admit men to practice. Meantime, the existence of reputable men in medicine as well as in law was assumed in the earliest references to "authorized Phisitians," and implied such preliminary *esprit de corps* as was necessary to the later founding of guild institutions. It was probably gentlemen of this superior type, a small group usually located in large towns, who provided later historians with favorable impressions of colonial practitioners.

At the instigation of this better class of medical men (in the early period, often clergymen) efforts had occasionally been made to require competence before granting formal approval to practice. This was in line with the original Massachusetts' Act of 1649: a law which in theory was also adopted in New York and New Jersey under the Duke of York code of 1665. Thus, in Boston, the Suffolk County Court, in the single year 1672, had granted one man permission to practice and fined another for proceeding without such approval. (Perhaps the latter action was another sign that Americans wished to go further than the British in punishing anyone who practiced without a license.) But such episodes were sporadic: there was no systematic procedure. Indeed, the man approved in 1672 owed his success to the testimony of those already his "grateful patients."[26]

Although no regulation was really attempted before the 1760s, it was not because educated men were indifferent to the problem. Just as the first law on the subject was passed in Massachusetts, so it was also in the Bay Colony that a striking appeal for control was made early in the next century. One surmises that, since this item has survived, similar ones may have been lost or were never printed. Indeed, the statement

[26] Carl Bridenbaugh, *Cities in the Wilderness* (New York: Ronald, 1938), p. 89; Packard, *History of Medicine* (n. 1, above), p. 170; Blanton, *Medicine in Virginia* (n. 2, above), p. 97; Spector, "The Growth of Medicine" (n. 16, above), pp. 513 f.

published in Boston, 1737–38, suggests that a few observers held strong convictions on this issue throughout the later colonial era, but always encountered indifference or opposition on the part of the majority. Most men seem to have believed that a people who entrusted their souls to all sorts of preachers, could likewise entrust their bodies to all sorts of "doctors."

The statement by one "Philanthropus" appeared in the *Boston Weekly Newsletter* and was addressed to the medical society in that city. This society, probably the first in the English colonies, had been formed during the 1730s to urge some regulation of practice. No doubt "Philanthropus" was a member. At any rate, he began by making the usual accusation that "we are infected with . . . an Infatuation in favour of Empiricism or Quackery"; and then reminded readers that although "our laws" do nothing about this, "the laws of England do":

> Our Ancestors did not think fit to rest the Safety of the Subjects upon . . . the Common Law alone, but have made several Acts of Parliament for regulating the Practice of Physick . . . .

After which, recalling the old statute incorporating the London College of Physicians and the methods used to enforce it, he continued:

> Methinks it would be . . . of no great Difficulty to concert some proper measures for regulating the Practice of Physick throughout this Province . . . so that no person shall be allowed to practice Physick within . . . this Province, unless he be first examined by such regular, approved . . . Physicians and Surgeons as the Honourable Court shall see meet to appoint.

Finally, anticipating sympathy for the popular man "of no learning"—a sentiment often expressed both before and after 1737—"Philanthropus" pointed out that such a practitioner could continue his calls "if upon examination [he] is found to understand his business." But if not, patients "are safer without him; and it's more prudent trusting to the care of Providence and a good Nurse than such a vile Imposture." One would now add a fervent amen, but the honourable court of the time was apparently unmoved.[27]

It may be remarked in passing, that "Philanthropus" clearly wished to prevent any ignorant person from practicing, even though the latter made no pretense to learning. Here again, Americans went beyond the British principle of *caveat emptor* in regard to medical services.

Local or provincial statements about midwifery were not uncommon but involved no strict controls. In 1738, for example, a law was adopted for "Regulating Midwives within the City of New York," but this was concerned chiefly with ethical matters and made no reference to examinations. The applicant was required, nevertheless, to "take the Oath of a Midwife," which was specific in regard to professional conduct at a time when "doctors" faced no tests whatever. Such a ceremony, held before and recorded by the highest authorities, may well have screened out the worst risks and presumably set apart women officially approved. In any case, the law testified to the esteem in which some "Midwives and expert Women in that Faculty" were still held at the time. It is also interesting that, only a decade before men began to invade obstetrical practice, the midwives of 1738 had to swear not to "open any mystery appertaining to your Office, in the presence of any Man, unless Necessity . . . constrain you to do so."[28]

The first native medical school—perhaps one should say the first British provincial school—was finally founded in Philadelphia in 1765. This institution might have grown up within the already-existing Pennsylvania Hospital if London examples had been followed, but it was modeled instead on Edinburgh in being affiliated with the arts faculty of the college which later became the University of Pennsylvania. Dr. John Morgan,

[27] *Boston Weekly News Letter,* January 5, 1737/38. See also Bridenbaugh, *Cities in the Wilderness* (n. 26, above), p. 403.
[28] *New York Weekly Journal,* June 26, 1738.

the founder, wished to train physicians to practice only in the best London tradition but, as noted, such open distinctions were ignored and indeed were unrealistic in the colonies. Morgan also hoped to found an elect College of Physicians which would hold examinations and grant licenses for the colonies as a whole. The proprietors were advised in London, however, that the Royal College there had exercised a monopoly and the Penns therefore refused to charter such an institution in Philadelphia.[29] Thus ended the first attempt to grant licensing powers to professional bodies in the British manner.

The requirement of governmental licenses, on the other hand, was first adopted in New York (for New York City) as early as 1760.[30] More significant were developments in New Jersey, where a provincial medical society was formed in 1766. This society was chiefly concerned with raising the standards and income of practitioners, and it soon requested the provincial government to set up a licensing system. The result was that, in 1772, the Legislature and Governor William Franklin (son of Benjamin) adopted an act to regulate medical practice throughout New Jersey. This statute related to "Physic and Surgery" and required that all persons wishing to practice should be examined and approved "by any two of the Judges of the Supreme Court"—the latter to be assisted by any persons they thought fit. Vestiges of guild distinctions survived in provisions that approval could be extended to a "Physician or Surgeon," or to "a Physician *and* Surgeon [in British terms, read 'or Surgeon-Apothecary'] as the case may be." Fines were

[29] W. J. Bell, Jr., *John Morgan* . . . (Philadelphia: Univ. of Penna. Press, 1965), pp. 137–40; R. H. Shryock, *Medicine and Society in America, 1660–1860* (New York: New York Univ. Press, 1960), pp. 26–30 (reprinted [paperback]; Ithaca: Cornell Univ. Press, 1960), pp. 26–30; G. W. Corner, *Two Centuries of Medicine* . . . (Philadelphia: Lippincott, 1965), chap. 2.

[30] The *New York Gazette,* June 16, 1760. H. E. Sigerist states that according to the law, "no one should practise medicine or surgery or both" without examination and license (*American Medicine,* n. 8, above), p. 45. The Act is quoted in B. Stookey, *A History of Colonial Medical Education in* . . . *New York* (Springfield, Ill.: Thomas, 1962), pp. 8 f.

to be imposed on those who practiced for fees without being licensed in this manner.[31] Little is known about the enforcement of the program, if any, but in principle the Act of 1772 set up a colonial prototype of the later state boards of medical examiners.

Soon after the New Jersey society was founded, a somewhat different effort was undertaken in Sharon, Litchfield County, Connecticut. In 1767 some thirty "doctors" there organized what was at first an entirely local body. It was apparently this same society which, in 1769, petitioned the provincial Legislature for authority to examine and license practitioners—a reassertion of the idea of professional control. The request aroused in the *Connecticut Courant* (Hartford) the usual debate between opponents who warned against monopoly, and those who wished to certify practitioners. When opponents stated that quacks were in any case too numerous to suppress, the petitioners defended certain persons so designated because "some of the best physicians in this colony . . . were never under the care of any particular tutor." It seems strange that reformers would approve men who had not even served apprenticeships, yet the society was confident it could somehow separate the sheep from the goats. Anyone who denied this possibility, the members declared, was "an enemy of physic and all learning."

The petition was read privately in Hartford but not brought up formally before the Assembly, which thus failed to grant the society a charter. The Litchfield group made a more serious attempt, however, than did a similar society at Norwich, which in 1763 actually voted down a proposal to request licensing powers. Moreover, the Litchfield society later renewed its

---

[31] S. Allinson, ed., *Acts of the General Assembly of the Province of New Jersey, 1702–1776* (XII George III, 1772) (Burlington, N.J.: 1776), italics inserted. See also D. L. Cowen, *Medicine and Health in New Jersey: A History* (Princeton: Princeton Univ. Press, 1964), pp. 10–14; F. B. Rogers and A. R. Sayre, *The Healing Art: A History of the New Jersey Medical Society* (New Jersey Med. Soc., 1966).

offensive. In 1770 its officers addressed an appeal to "the Public" and announced that doctors from neighboring provinces had now become members. No doubt this came about because Sharon was close to the boundaries of both New York and Massachusetts, and one notes here the only interprovincial medical society on record. It apparently ceased to be active soon thereafter, however, for the last notice of its meetings for some years appeared in *The Courant* on November 19, 1771.[32]

The growing crisis with the mother country during the 70s diverted interests into political channels. The Revolution which began in 1776 doubtless delayed the formation of both local and state medical societies, but it benefited medical men in at least one respect. War brought "doctors" together from many areas for military service, and this in turn led—on Dr. John Morgan's recommendation—to attempts to assure standards among them by qualifying examinations. The procedure became routine and probably encouraged later demands for such tests in civilian practice.[33]

As prospects for independence improved, moreover, medical men shared in the resulting enthusiasm. If the United States were to become a nation coequal with others—a nation which might even offer new hope for all mankind—should not medicine share in this alluring future? Could there not be independence in art and science as well as in political life? Such anticipation transformed earlier confidence in local practice into pride in American medicine as a whole. Such pride, by the early 1800s, reached a state bordering on euphoria. All this was a bit premature—by a century or more—but the enthusiasm did infuse some vigor into professional activities. Moreover, it enabled doctors to identify professional advances with

[32] B. Stookey, "Found! The Record of the 1767 Medical Society in Litchfield," *Jour. Conn. State Med. Soc.,* XXI (March, 1957), 192, 347–52.

[33] Brooke Hindle, *The Pursuit of Science in Revolutionary America, 1735–1789* (Chapel Hill: Univ. of N.C. Press, 1956), p. 236.

national progress and so to appeal for what had hitherto been lacking; namely, popular support for medical reform.

In this respect doctors were more fortunate at first than lawyers; for the latter, having established some prestige by the 1760s, suffered in reputation after the Revolution because of services rendered to Tories seeking to recover lost property. Lawyers regained ground by 1800, however, by which time most states boasted some requirements for apprenticeship training (clerkships). Somewhat earlier, meanwhile, the states began to call for standards in medical education. It was probably more than coincidence that what is often viewed as the first law school was set up, about 1783, in the same Litchfield County which had already produced an ambitious medical society.[34]

An expression of real *élan* among doctors appeared in what may have been a revival of this same Litchfield group. On July 5, 1779, some two years before the end of actual combat, an ostensibly new group was formed at Sharon with the resounding title of "The first Medical Society in the thirteen United States of America." Dr. James Potter, once president of the earlier society, assumed the same post in the new organization—a body which continued the tradition of interstate membership. In 1780 it moved its headquarters to New Fairfield, where it survived for two or three more years. Like most later societies, it encouraged an *esprit de corps* and endured orations on science, ethics, and professional income. Following British tradition, its members foreswore all connections with "vain pretenders to physic" (irregulars). Moreover, having failed in the earlier appeal to Hartford, the society now set up its own procedures for examining candidates who desired approval. Even their own members—upon motion of any two

---

[34] Shryock, *Medicine and Society* (n. 29, above), pp. 117–19, concerning medicine. On the legal trends, see J. A. Krout and D. R. Fox, *The Completion of Independence, 1790–1830* (New York: Macmillan, 1944), pp. 279 f., 283.

colleagues—could be subjected to what amounted to re-examination.[35]

The most striking address heard in New Fairfield was that presented by Dr. Potter, in 1780, in which he emphasized an idea still novel among Americans: the value of research. Unlike Cotton Mather, who in 1724 had admitted the lack of science in the colonies, Potter agreed with Franklin that the time was at hand when Americans could be original as well as practical. Dr. Morgan, in 1765, had noted the need for investigations, and several native doctors had published clinical papers abroad, but few had approached the vision which thrilled the leader in rural Connecticut:

> The learning of all nations and ages, [Potter declared] is con centrated in America . . . . Therefore, strain every nerve . . . and push your researches with relentless impetuosity, through physics vast and ample field; . . . while you rest secure under the glorious, sacred and permanent independence of America.[36]

Naive as this peroration seems, Dr. Potter here invoked the very influence which would in time upgrade all medical education and licensure.

Small as it was, "the first Medical Society in the thirteen United States" took one other step, made possible by political upheavals. Despite its assumption of licensing powers, the society never forgot that even self-regulation would be more secure if given official approval. But having once been rebuffed

[35] References to the Litchfield societies are listed in F. Guerra's *American Medical Bibliography, 1639–1783* (New York: Lathrop Harper, 1962), p. 484, *passim.* See the *Connecticut Courant* . . . (Hartford: October 26, 1779); and W. B. McDaniel, II, "A Brief Sketch of the Rise of American Medical Societies," in F. Marti-Ibanez, ed., *History of American Medicine: A Symposium* (New York: M.D. Publications, 1958), p. 136.

[36] Potter's *Oration* (Hartford: Hudson and Goodwin, 1781), is noted in the bibliographies of Evans (no. 17315), and of R. B. Austin (no. 1557), and is reproduced in Shipton's microcard series. See also B. Hindle, *Science in Revolutionary America* (n. 33, above), p. 112. In this *Oration,* noted in the studies by W. B. McDaniel, II, of early American medical historiography, Potter stated that he had given an oration at Litchfield "fourteen years earlier" [1766] on the general history of medicine.

by a provincial legislature it decided to overlook British precedents and to seek advice from France—a new-found ally. Dr. Potter therefore prepared, in 1780, a formal appeal to the Royal Society of Medicine in Paris requesting moral support and guidance. The memorandum was sent to Franklin—then American minister to France—with the request that he translate it and see that it received due consideration.[37] There is no evidence of what happened thereafter, yet this appeal to national authorities, bypassing Hartford completely, makes one wonder whether the society hoped to secure some sort of federal charter from the Continental Congress. If so, the incident was probably a unique exception to the native tradition of provincial/state controls. The Articles of Confederation would hardly have sanctioned such an affront to "sovereign states," but perhaps Dr. Potter was already a potential federalist. In any case he was moved not only by patriotic, pro-French ardor but also by an invincible faith in the "Progress of Physic in America."

The society at New Fairfield never, in itself, exercised much influence and yet it illustrated the alternatives confronting professional men at the advent of independence. Here was a local society which was simultaneously a tristate body, and which was even more *outré* in aspiring to foreign contacts. Such contacts, moreover, were to be with France rather than Britain, anticipating French influence in American medicine which did not actually take form until four decades thereafter.

The demise of this imaginative group did not check the founding of local societies, but it did show that even the Revolution could not change basic professional patterns. The ulti-

---

[37] My colleague, Dr. W. J. Bell, Jr., called my attention to the letter of James Potter, President, New Fairfield, Conn., May 10, 1780, to Benjamin Franklin, in Paris, enclosing formal appeal to the Royal French Society; Franklin Papers, Amer. Phil. Soc., Misc., vol. 54, pt. 1, Folios 1–72, pp. 67 f. See also Hindle, *Science in Revolutionary America* (n. 33, above), p. 292. Professor L. W. Labaree informs me that no reply from Franklin or from the French Society has been found.

mate authority to license, as indicated in New Jersey, was to remain with the states rather than with voluntary or with national agencies. Meantime, British traditions rather than French would be taken for granted for some time to come.

Within a year after the New Fairfield appeal to Franklin, a state medical society was organized in Massachusetts, and as soon as the war ended, other such bodies began to appear along the seaboard. By 1815 societies had been founded in most of the original thirteen states and by 1830 in nearly all the states of the Union. Each of these organizations advocated tests and licensing, and in most cases legislatures responded in some measure. N. S. Davis later stated that by the 1830s only three states—Pennsylvania, Virginia, and North Carolina – lacked such statutes. These acts were state-wide in coverage but varied widely in other respects. In some cases, state examining boards were created. In other instances, state medical societies were granted power to test and license, and this might be done by one central board or by censors chosen for particular counties or districts. The testing was done largely if not exclusively by medical men, usually in the form of oral quizzes which must have differed from state to state, or county to county.

Somewhat similar trends appeared in the legal field, where various societies were founded in the chief cities between 1789 and 1820. After the latter date, several state bar associations were established—as in Mississippi in 1824, and in Kentucky in 1847. Both the local and state bodies desired laws on training by apprenticeship, and some formal education was available in a few law schools founded before 1830. By 1800, fifteen of the nineteen states had nominal rules for admission to practice. Yet, except in Massachusetts, little real control was attained. The legal profession was, at best, no more successful than the medical in providing regulations.

A closer look at medical developments makes it clear that the era 1780–1830 was one of uncertainty about both ends and means. In a country where virtually no oversight over medical practice had been exercised before 1780, decisions had to be made among a number of alternatives; to wit, state or voluntary (society) regulations; penalties or no action in case of violations; central or local administration; exclusive licensing by a state body or a sharing of this power with the schools; and finally, whether to exempt men already in practice from these procedures?

Decisions on the last question were similar in most cases. Men already in practice were exempt from new regulations; and so likewise, as a rule, were "doctors" who had been in good standing in other states. Such reciprocity was almost taken for granted at a time when regulations were flexible or difficult to enforce.

Although there was no uniformity, most states acceded to the wishes of medical societies in delegating licensing authority to these bodies. New Jersey, which began in 1772 by setting up a single government board, in 1790 authorized the state medical society to take over this power and to act through district units. New York, which had begun with a state-appointed board in 1760, switched to a system similar to that of New Jersey in 1806. Alabama was exceptional when, in 1823, it provided five district boards elected by the Legislature. But from the start, most New England states and also those of the "Old Northwest" (Ohio, Indiana, Michigan) placed licensing powers in the hands of state or local medical societies.

In this trend there was adherence to the British tradition of voluntary controls, but in the matter of penalties for enforcement the states continued to diverge from British toward European usage in attempts to ban all quackery. In a few instances, such as South Carolina in 1817, it is not clear whether the state medical society could penalize unlicensed men, but in most cases the societies could bring action against "quacks"—usually in the county courts for moderate fines. Prohibitions were occasionally quite specific; for example, in New Jersey, acts of 1813 and 1818 required the suppression of "all irregular bred contenders . . . under the names . . . of practicing botanists, root or Indian doctors . . . or any other quacks." Usually, penalties were permitted only when a man charged for his services, since home remedies and "kitchen physic" were commonly employed and generally approved—at least for minor illness. It was in this connection that New York, perhaps unwittingly, encouraged quackery by exempting all persons using "native vegetable drugs" from the application of the licensing laws.[38]

The problem of whether medical schools as well as societies could issue licenses first appeared in Massachusetts, where the state medical society was authorized in 1781 to examine candidates without reference to guild distinctions. The first men so examined—like most of the examiners—had been trained only by apprenticeships. After the Harvard medical school was founded in 1783, however, the question arose: Should any further examination be required of its graduates? The medical society at first insisted on its right to pass on every man who desired certification—with or without a degree. Under pressure, however, a public examination was held of all candidates, and the Harvard M.D.s so outshone the others that licenses could not be long refused to such men. After 1803 *either* the Harvard diploma or examination by the society qualified a man

---

[38] C. B. Coventry, "History of Medical Legislation in the State of New York," *N.Y. Jour. of Med.,* IV (1845), 152. N. S. Davis, *Medical Education and Medical Institutions in the U.S.A., 1776-1876* (Washington: U.S. Bureau of Education, 1877), pp. 51–56. On South Carolina, see J. I.Waring, *A History of Medicine in South Carolina* (Charleston: S.C. Med. Assoc., 1964), pp. 118 ff., 160. See also J. F. Kett, "Regulation of the Medical Profession in America, 1780–1860," unpublished thesis, Harvard University, 1964.

for practice.[39] Here was further conformity to British precedent.

This dual system was subsequently followed in several other states, for example, by Connecticut in 1810 and by South Carolina in 1817. In the first of these instances an unusual arrangement was made in that candidates were examined by a joint board representing the state medical society and the medical faculty of Yale College. Licenses were granted by the society after one course of lectures (of four months) at the college, and degrees were awarded by Yale after two courses. But the Carolina Legislature adopted what soon became the common rule, that is, tests *could* be held by the state society but graduation from any chartered medical school was all that was needed in order to practice. Georgia is said to have gone so far in 1821 as to require an M.D. of all future practitioners. Theoretically, such a demand could have been met by degrees granted by medical societies as well as by schools, and this experiment was actually made in New Jersey. In that state, which had an unusual record in licensing matters, the state society was authorized in 1825 to grant the M.D. degree. This title was given sporadically until 1902, sometimes after an examination, sometimes as an honorary award.[40]

Apparently, a medical degree impressed American legislatures more during the era after 1780 than did an apprenticeship followed only by an examination before a state board or society. One can understand this in view of several circumstances: first, apprenticeship was often casual and inadequate;

[39] Josiah Bartlett, . . . *Progress of Medical Science in . . . Massachusetts* (Boston: 1810), pp. 15–25; H. R. Viets, *A Brief History of Medicine in Massachusetts* (Boston: Houghton-Mifflin, 1930), pp. 120 ff.; Hindle, *Science in Revolutionary America* (n. 33, above), p. 291; W. A. Burrage, *A History of the Massachusetts Medical Society* (Boston: privately printed, 1923), pp. 302 f., 316.

[40] On South Carolina, see Waring, *Medicine in South Carolina* (n. 38, above), p. 160; on Connecticut, W. J. Bell, Jr., "The Medical Institution of Yale College, 1810–1885," *Yale Jour. of Biol. and Med.*, vol. 33 (1960), pp. 170–73; on New Jersey, F. B. Rogers, "Medical Doctor's Degree Given by Medical Society of New Jersey," *Jour. Med. Soc. of N.J.*, vol. 53 (1956), p. 327.

second, most of the early faculties—the seven founded before 1810—maintained reasonably good standards; and, finally, since the schools provided little clinical training, they all required apprenticeship for admission. In other words, their students shared with non-graduates the uncertain values of apprenticeship and also obtained formal education.

Prospects for licensing therefore seemed promising in the early 1800s, especially to older men who could recall the days when there had been no controls whatever. In nearly all states, candidates were supposed to pass examinations either within the schools or before state boards or societies. It is true that the ancient specialty of midwifery was subject at best to only casual regulation, perhaps because "doctors" were by that time taking over most obstetrical practice among the upper classes. Hence, midwives (who continued to practice among the poor) lost the status enjoyed by some colonial predecessors. It is also true that sheer quackery flourished as never before, but this was also the case abroad, and American authorities, like the French and the German, failed in attempts to ban such practice by legislation.[41]

Unfortunately, the promise of early American laws proved illusory, and for half a century after 1820 licensing requirements apparently deteriorated. By the 1850s, when German authorities were establishing uniform standards and when the British government was taking the first steps toward national control, the situation in the United States seemed to be approaching its nadir. Explanations of this contrast are complex but may be summarized briefly.

[41] American quackery of this era is analyzed in James H. Young's *Toadstool Millionaires* (Princeton: Princeton Univ. Press, 1961). On the German experience, see H. Magnus, *Die Kurierfreiheit, u. das Recht auf den eignen Körper: Ein geschichtlicher Beitrag zum Kampf gegen das Kurpfuschertum* (Breslau: 1905), pp. 1–4; on France, G. Bourgeau, *Les Erreurs de la grande Presse en Matière Médicale* (Paris: 1916), pp. 37–39. See also J. H. Young's analysis in "American Medical Quackery in the Age of the Common Man," *Miss. Valley Hist. Rev.*, XLVII (March, 1961) 579–93.

In the first place, the very prestige accorded early medical colleges encouraged deterioration. When degrees were accepted as superior licenses more and more candidates desired them on the easiest possible terms. In response, new institutions were founded after 1810, and at a growing rate after 1840. Twenty-six were set up between 1810 and 1840, and forty-seven between 1840 and 1875. (These figures do not include various private institutes, in such fields as anatomy and surgery, which were maintained by hospital staff members in the chief medical centers.) Professors in these schools, however genuine their ideals, were paid directly by student fees, and they were often tempted to lower requirements so as to secure as many students as possible. Competition with rival colleges, also seeking large classes, increased this temptation. Even more disturbing was the advent of schools owned and operated by doctors, primarily for profit. Beginning as early as 1812 in Maryland, legislatures were persuaded to charter proprietary colleges which were affiliated neither with arts faculties (as in Edinburgh) nor with hospitals (as in London).[42] Parenthetically, real hospital schools of the London type did not appear until the 1860s, with the founding of Bellevue in New York City and the Long Island College in Brooklyn.

To make matters worse, sectarian colleges—homeopathic, eclectic, "botanic"—invaded the country after 1830 and did battle with "regular" schools of any type. Obviously, ill-informed legislatures still thought one sort of medical practice as promising as another: a practical and equalitarian people could decide for themselves which type was most effective.

[42] W. F. Norwood, *Medical Education in the United States Before the Civil War* (Philadelphia: Univ. of Penna. Press, 1944), p. 430; Davis, *Medical Education and Medical Institutions* (n. 38, above), p. 41. For critical German opinion of both American and British medical education, see T. Puschmann, *A History of Medical Education,* trans. E. H. Hare (London: Lewis, 1891), pp. 449–506. See also Norwood's summary article "American Medical Education from the Revolutionary War to the Civil War," *Jour. Med. Educ.,* vol. 32 (June, 1957), pp. 433–47.

When doctors protested against irregular practice they were accused of seeking a monopoly for their own benefit. Dr. N. S. Davis later claimed that the sects invented this accusation after 1840, in their crusade for medical freedom as analogous to religious freedom, but the evidence for earlier distrust of monopoly is clear enough. The sectarians doubtless stirred up old fears, condemning what they now termed "orthodox intolerance." Moreover, the more learned sects—homeopathy and eclecticism—could then make a better plea for heresy on medical grounds than was to be the case a few decades later.[43]

There had been those in the United Kingdom who likewise decried monopolies, for this was supposedly the great era of laissez faire, but in Britain old institutions came down from a time when monopoly had been more or less respectable and so these corporations could continue to exercise some influence. In its negative aspect the American situation reflected the absence of such traditional restraints as well as the lack of any national control.

Scientific claims made for new schools were supplemented by economic pleas. Was there not a need for low-cost colleges which would give poor boys a chance to practice? And what of costs to patients? Sectarians held that a monopoly for regulars would limit the number of doctors and so increase fees— a conspiracy in restraint of trade. Meantime, many persons assumed that the proliferation of schools was a response to population expansion. How else could the profession keep in step with the number of patients? This justification for obscure faculties seemed plausible, but overlooked the fact that population increases in western Europe resulted in no such cheapening of medical education.

[43] R. H. Shryock, "Public Relations of the Medical Profession in Great Britain and the United States: 1600–1870," *Annals of Med. Hist.*, n. s., Vol. 2 (1930), pp. 318–23; also Shryock, *Medicine and Society* (n. 29, above), pp. 144–46; and Alex Berman, "Neo-Thomsonianism in the United States," *Bull. Hist. of Med.*, XI (1956), 133–55.

Also overlooked was the ratio of "doctors" to population, which had long seemed higher in the United States than abroad. Hence professional leaders were convinced that, despite population growth, too many graduates were being turned out each year. Various factors influenced this doctor-patient ratio then as they do now. In 1850, for example, definitions were involved. American estimates included under "physicians" all who held any sort of M.D., and probably others as well, whereas European nations may have omitted their second-class men. If so, the latter countries had more "doctors" in the American sense than the statistics showed. Nevertheless, cumulative evidence indicates a continuing excess of practitioners in America until after 1910.[44]

Professional leaders in "the States," at first proud of their new schools and regulations, became disillusioned by the 1820s. In 1826, for example, the president of the New York State Medical Society warned that bargain degrees were already offered which required less of students than did the examinations given those trained only by apprenticeship. Meanwhile, despite such warnings, it appeared that certain states—chiefly those west of the Appalachians—just left it to their citizens to seek out M.D.s and enacted no licensing laws whatever. By 1845 there were at least eight such states in the Union, and some ten others had repealed earlier regulations. In Georgia, and perhaps a few other states, examining boards continued a legal existence but graduates of chartered medical colleges could ignore them. It was reported in 1849 that only New Jersey and the District of Columbia retained any real control of licensure. In apparent desperation a pro-

[44] In 1900, e.g., the ratio in the United States was estimated at about 1:600; in the United Kingdom at 1:1,100; J. R. Patterson, "Professional Education," in N.M. Butler, ed., *Education in the United States* (Albany: Lyon, 1900), p. 54. See also S. E. Harris, *The Economics of American Medicine* (New York: Macmillan, 1964), pp. 107–14.

posal was made that national (federal) licenses be provided, but this was unrealistic at the time.[45]

Similar deterioration could be observed in the legal field, as the states repealed or neglected to enforce earlier controls over practice. By 1840 only eleven of thirty states maintained regulations for admission to the bar. Lawyers, like doctors, were accused of monopolies and there were demands for abolishing the legal profession altogether.[46] This attitude suggests vestiges of colonial suspicion and of the ire aroused during the Revolution—old resentments directed more against law than against medicine. Both professions, however, suffered from the individualism and anti-intellectualism associated with Jacksonian democracy.

Anti-intellectualism, like Jacksonian democracy, is of course defined in different ways and subject to diverse interpretations. In the case of lawyers and doctors, their possession of "learning" (which could be used to exploit laymen) was one cause of suspicion which might be termed anti-intellectualism. On the other hand, few doctors and lawyers could have been accused of being "intellectuals," as the term is now used. One can realize this in the case of medical men by noting the educational background of a large sample of the profession.

In 1850 an astute doctor checked the qualifications of practitioners in eastern Tennessee. In that area, 201 "physicians" served a population of 164,000. Of these men 35 (only 17 per cent) were graduates of some sort of regular school; 42 (20 per cent) said they had "taken one course of lectures" but

---

[45] See *Transactions of the New York State Med. Soc. for the Years 1807–1831* (Albany: 1868), pp. 350 f. (1826). For the origins and later breakdown in licensing codes in four states, 1780–1850, see Kett, "Regulation of the Medical Profession" (n. 38, above). On the early proposal for a federal license, see the *N.Y. Jour. of Med.,* V (1845), 415.

[46] C. B. Coventry, "History of Medical Legislation in the State of New York," *N.Y. Jour. of Med.,* IV (1845), 152–61. See also *Boston Med. and Surg. Jour.,* XXVIII (1843), 523; *Trans.,* AMA (1849), pp. 326 ff. On lawyers, see Chroust, *Legal Profession in America* (n. 5, above), pp. 137–69, 288.

had not graduated; and 27 (13 per cent) were "botanic and steamers." Most of the others (almost 50 per cent) had received no instruction other than "reading, which for the most part was limited."[47] Some of the latter group must have been pretenders; others doubtless had been denied formal training by poverty and isolation. Qualifications were presumably better in large towns, but the American population was still dominantly rural at the time.

How uncontrolled practice was by the 1830s is best illustrated by the rise of medical sects without pretense to learning. The most successful empirics were the "botanic doctors" mentioned above—sometimes termed Thomsonians after their founder "Doctor" S. A. Thomson. The latter evolved his own form of practice, which condemned the use of calomel (mercury) as a purgative and revived an old dependence on vegetable drugs.

Thomson displayed some imagination in patenting his "system" and in selling rights to employ it. As a licensing program, this scheme was unique in its open commercialism and in the control exercised by one man. What proportion of the botanic doctors had merely read the founder's writings, and how many had had other forms of training, is not clear; in any case, they were usually able to practice at will. Like the homeopaths, they formed societies and so confronted the regulars with an organized, rival profession. All this occurred after 1838, however, by which time—as Dr. Alex Berman has pointed out—most "botanics" had broadened their practice and were no longer loyal to Thompson's teachings.

In contrast to the ease with which educational standards could be by-passed in entering practice, racial barriers were insurmountable. Free, elementary schooling was available to

[47] Philip M. Hamer, ed., *The Centennial History of the Tennessee State Medical Association* (Nashville: 1930), pp. 22 f. On anti-intellectualism in general, see Merle Curti, "Intellectuals and Other People," *Amer. Hist. Rev.,* LX (January, 1955), 261–73.

colored children in northern cities, but the issue of admitting Negroes to medical schools does not seem to have arisen before 1865. In the South slave or free Negroes occasionally acquired reputations as healers, and slave women served as midwives, but such activities did not constitute general participation in practice. The situation was quite different from that in Spanish America, where national *protomédicatos* failed in attempts to exclude mulattoes or *mestizos* from formal education and practice. On the other hand, as Professor John T. Lanning has shown, Spanish-American authorities made it difficult for illegitimate persons to become physicians or surgeons. In this regard, Anglo-Americans were more liberal.

It is clear, whatever their social background, that many "doctors" in the United States were second-grade men in a professional sense. As will be noted, it was assumed by some observers that such men were needed to look after the poor. But most Americans, in the absence of open distinctions, probably thought that they were cared for by real physicians. It might have been safer, or at least more candid, to have given many of these "docs" some lesser title.

It was during the 1840s, under these circumstances, that professional leaders finally attempted to bring order out of chaos. It so happened that national medical and scientific societies were formed in most European countries between 1820 and 1860, in response to scientific progress and to improved means for communication. In the medical world these bodies—e.g., the Provincial Medical and Surgical Association in England (1832)—represented all regular practitioners rather than any one guild. The need for a similar, voluntary society was clear in the United States, particularly in view of the indifference of the federal government to medical affairs. Proposals were made as early as the 1830s to form a national organization, and one wonders whether French reforms may have suggested these early American efforts to set up some central body. On the other hand, Gallic influence usually related more to science than to professional matters. Centralization in French administration was actually at the opposite pole from American decentralization, and it seems more probable that it was still the British tradition which inspired American developments. At any rate, it was not until 1846—in response to a call from the New York State Medical Society—that a preliminary meeting made plans for founding the American Medical Association (A.M.A.), in 1847.

The immediate occasion of the New York invitation was a protest against permitting professors to license their own students—particularly when the latter might expect this reward in return for fees. (Not until after 1860 did the University of Michigan and one or two other state institutions begin to pay salaries to medical professors in the German manner.) As early as 1839 the New York society had protested the combination of teaching and licensing powers, and it maintained this position in hoping that a national body might bring about a separation of the two functions. In other words, this society—even as other strong state and local units—viewed the deterioration of the medical schools with alarm and wished to bring them under professional control.[48]

The national association represented only "regular" societies and schools, and hoped to influence state authorities on behalf of the public as well as of the profession. But its programs for sanitary codes and vital statistics were secondary to the desire to raise educational and licensing standards. Unfortunately, there was a built-in obstacle here in the composition of the

[48] See N. S. Davis, *Medical Education and Medical Institutions* (n. 38, above), p. 47. The official records of the AMA are given in Morris Fishbein's *A History of the American Medical Association, 1847–1947* (Philadelphia: 1947). For the later AMA history, see J. G. Burrow, *AMA: Voice of American Medicine* (Baltimore: The Johns Hopkins Press, 1963); also D. E. Konold, *A History of American Medical Ethics* (Madison: State Hist. Soc. of Wis., 1962), pp. 16–18.

association itself. Many of its members held vested interests in weak colleges and the licenses provided by their degrees. Such "professors" blocked any statement on standards for apprenticeship, and defeated all efforts to exclude representation of faculties as such. Within each state, moreover, these men exerted influence on politicians in the interest of inferior colleges. Some leaders from the better schools rose above this level, but their political effectiveness within states was limited; nor could they, in the American setting, appeal for control through national legislation. There could be little reform under these circumstances.[49]

Indeed, matters grew worse after 1850, with the proliferation of sectarian colleges. Although certain of these were more or less respectable, many were not. In the early 1860s, for example, a "Doctor" T. H. Trall secured a charter for his water-cure institute in New York City. Thereafter, he could bestow the M.D. degree on those who followed his lectures on hydropathy, Grahamism, vegetarianism, and the like. Yet even so bizarre an institution may have had merits lacking in low-grade, regular schools. Some light is thrown on these commercialized colleges by the letters of Dr. Richard Arnold of Savannah, a graduate of Princeton and of the University of Pennsylvania medical school who was devoted to reform. In 1857, for example, he wrote a New York colleague that:

> We have taken the first bold, unequivocal stand against a growing abuse, viz. taking a winter student, hurrying him through a Summer Course and turning him out a Doctor in less than a year. . . . This has been done by Oglethorpe College here . . . . The Atlanta College avows and defends this course . . . . When schools can act in this

[49] A committee "on teaching and licensing," appointed at a preliminary meeting in 1846, offered majority and minority reports in 1847. The former made no specific suggestions, the latter merely proposed that state society representatives "sit in" with college examiners. The 1847 convention took no action on either report. See *Proceedings of the National Medical Conventions* . . . (Philadelphia: AMA, 1847), pp. 37, 107 ff., 114 ff.

way . . . are we not falling upon evil days? As God is my judge I speak for the Profession at large and not for our college.[50]

The low level of medical education in the era 1830–80 was reflected not only in the schools but also in the reputation of their students. The public image of such students had been none too high in Europe, and in England some professors as well as their classes had a reputation for crudity.[51] But opinion of American students, as expressed in the newspapers in the training centers, was sometimes extreme in its disdain. In 1858, for example, the Philadelphia *City Item* declared that these men were coarse and ignorant.[52] More colorful were the opinions of the New York *Sun* concerning Southern students in 1861, although these can be ascribed in part to sectional prejudice. An individual of this type, observed an editor, "is a long-haired, lantern-jawed verdant youth afflicted with chronic salivation and inveterate profanity . . . deriving his ideas of morals, grammer and behavior from his negro nurse . . . he becomes in New York a puzzle to professors, a terror to landladies, and a munificent patron of grog shops."[53]

Such comments suggest exaggeration but had some basis in fact. Criticism, moreover, was aimed not only at students: there was evidence of a low opinion of medical men in general. For although many persons maintained faith in family doctors, and some foreign travelers praised the profession in large cities,

[50] Shryock, ed., *Letters of Richard D. Arnold, M.D., 1808–1876* (Durham: Duke University Press, 1929), pp. 82 f. On indifference of some "regulars" to suppressing quackery, see T. N. Bonner, *Medicine in Chicago, 1850–1950* (Madison: Amer. Hist. Res. Center, 1957), pp. 13 f., 206; and on Trall, Shryock, "Sylvester Graham . . .," *Miss. Valley Hist. Rev.*, vol. 18 (September, 1931), pp. 180 ff.

[51] Newman, *Evolution of Medical Education* (n. 16, above), pp. 41–46. In contrast, the English traveler J. S. Buckingham declared in 1841 that New York doctors were "a more moral and religious body of men than . . . the same profession in . . . Europe," *America: Historical, Statistical, & Descriptive* (London: Fisher, 1841), I, 187 f.

[52] November 6, 1858.

[53] *Savannah Med. Jour.*, II (1861), 379 f. For a general discussion of American medical students, see G. W. Corner, *Proc. Amer. Phil. Soc.*, vol. 109, no. 5 (October, 1965).

widespread distrust also appeared and was at times deplored by physicians themselves. Newspapers carried accounts of bungled cases and lectured physicians on scientific problems. Occasionally, editors claimed that doctors tried to keep patients ill, or even indicted the entire profession as a "stupendous humbug."[54] The origins of this distrust have been mentioned—the emergence of medical sects, the general attitude of laissez faire, and the lack of such traditional restraints as were exercised in Europe by universities and guild corporations. Moreover, equalitarian sentiments were stronger by 1850 than they had been in 1750, and the masses had become more confident by the latter era that they could judge scientific matters for themselves.

State schools for example, had made the public literate enough to read attacks on "regulars," but not sufficiently educated to make discriminating judgments. As noted, moreover, the superiority of orthodox medicine still lay to some extent in the general education of its leaders rather than in any therapeutic advantage. Indeed, the mild practice of homeopaths was probably safer than that followed by regulars—though equally ineffective. Under these circumstances legislators chartered all sorts of medical schools, accepted cheap or even fraudulent diplomas, and left it to laymen to decide which type of practice was most helpful.

The difficulties which medicine as well as law confronted in an equalitarian society were well illustrated in the field which concerned both; that is, in forensic medicine or medical jurisprudence. Somewhat reminiscent of de Tocqueville's general comments on American society was a statement made by

[54] See, e.g., L. Bauer, "On the Declining Relations of the Medical Profession to the Public," *Cincinnati Medical Observer*, II (1857), 106; Paul F. Eve, "To What Cause Are We to Attribute the Diminished Respectability of the Medical Profession in the Estimation of the American Public?", *Medical and Surgical Reporter*, n.s., I (1858), 141, 143; *Harper's Weekly*, February 5, 1859; Elmira (N.Y.) *Daily Gazette*, May 20, 1879. For a favorable account of New York City doctors about 1840, however, see Buckingham, *America* (n. 51, above).

Dr. S. E. Chaillé of New Orleans at Philadelphia in 1876, concerning this aspect of law. Its application, he declared:

> varies with the appreciation of medical knowledge by the rulers of a nation; and (since an adequate appreciation is limited to the educated few, and is not yet disseminated among the mass of any people), it results, that laws more favorable to the culture of legal medicine are to be found in nations ruled by the educated few, than in those governed by the people.

But Chaillé then quoted Blackstone to the effect that backwardness in such matters was the price "free nations" paid for "liberty in more substantial matters."[55]

British as well as German experience in medical licensure after 1850 seemed to support Chaillé's views on the particular theme of forensic medicine. In contrast to seeming deterioration in "the States," the British made some progress toward medical reform in the famous Act of 1858. Two decades of agitation had preceded this legislation, much as demands for reform had anticipated early programs of the American Medical Association, but the outcomes were at first quite different in the two cases.[56] The Act of 1858 continued to leave licensing authority in the universities and in the old corporations and did not outlaw quackery or sectarianism as such, but it set up a National Registry of regular practitioners (those licensed by traditional bodies) and so identified the respectable personnel. The latter were granted privileges denied to others, such as the rights to sue for fees and to enter government service.

---

[55] Shryock, *Medicine and Society* (n. 29, above), pp. 142–49. See also Chaillé, "Origin and Progress of Medical Jurisprudence, 1776–1876" (1879), reprinted in *Jour. of Criminal Law . . .*, vol. 40, Nov. 1949, p. 398.

[56] How chaotic the British situation had still been during these decades was indicated in the general periodicals, e.g., "Medical Reform," *Edinburgh Rev.*, LXXXI (1845), 237 ff. In 1838 William Farr demanded a general reform of education and licensing and even urged the suppression of quackery, see his *British Medical Almanac* (London: 1838), pp. 175–79. A decade later a "National Institute of General Practitioners" had been formed and adopted a statement urging reform, see the *Report* of their Council, London, 1848. Also see Sir J. Simon, *English Sanitary Institutions* (London: 1897), p. 269.

The registry was maintained by a Council for Medical Education responsible to the Privy Council, and the former even had a right to modify examinations given by licensing bodies. In practice, however, it displayed restraint in not interfering with private institutions. Such restraint had merit in permitting self-improvement in schools and corporations, during which process professional bodies encouraged the adjustment of curricula and examinations to progress in medical science. These voluntary adjustments took time, however, and for some decades there was continuing disparity in the requirements of the dozen or more licensing bodies.[57] Reformers hoped to set up a single portal of entry into the profession, or at least to provide single examining boards for England, for Scotland, and for Ireland.

Although neither of these goals was fully attained, steps were finally taken toward a merger of certain licensing authorities. In 1884 the medical council approved the formation of a conjoint board, agreed upon by the Royal Colleges of Physicians and of Surgeons in London, as an examining body for granting admission to the National Registry.[58] This merger omitted the Society of Apothecaries, but the latter's L.S.A. (Licentiate Society of Apothecaries) authorized practice in both medicine and surgery. Meantime, the Royal College of Physicians of Edinburgh, in association with the College of Surgeons there and with the Faculty of Physicians and Surgeons of Glasgow, granted a double qualification which conferred the right to practice all branches of medicine throughout the United Kingdom. In 1884 the three Scottish bodies agreed to confer

[57] For continued difficulties and the need for further legislation as late as the 1880s, see William Dale, *The State of the Medical Profession of Great Britain and Ireland* (Dublin: Atkinson, 1875), pp. 9–84; H. J. Hardwick, *Medical Education and Practice in All Parts of the World* (London: 1880); T. H. Huxley, "The State of the Medical Profession," *The Nineteenth Century*, no. 84 (1884), pp. 228–38.

[58] Newman, *Evolution of Medical Education* (n. 16, above), chap. 6.

a triple qualification which indicated that its holders were licentiates of each of these institutions.[59]

Some consolidation in British procedures was thus attained at the very time when, as will be noted, about forty state licensing boards were set up in the American Union. In this respect, the British—taking off, as it were, from the Act of 1858—were in advance of Americans in efforts to standardize licensing procedures. It was not by chance, therefore, that when a voluntary national board was eventually formed in the United States, its founders looked in part to England and Scotland for guidance.

In respect to improvements within the schools, however, the British encountered difficulties similar to those experienced by Americans. Curiously enough, both countries seemed to share the very advantage said to account for the upsurge in German science after 1850. This was the existence of free, competing universities, in the absence of such centralized control as obtained in France. These apparent resemblances were superficial, however, until almost the end of the century. Competition in England was inhibited by what has been termed the "Oxford-Cambridge duopoly"—though this may not have explained Scottish trends—and in the United States there were no real universities in existence before 1875.

The whole contrast between scientific progress in the English- and in German-speaking countries was, indeed, quite complex and involved more than competition between universities. The British, responding slowly to basic research and specialization, neglected these procedures in the old universities and left it to individuals to become first-rate scientists, whereas the Germans centered science in university programs, systematically training not only first-rate but also second- and third-rate men who did

[59] I am indebted to Dr. H. P. Tait of Edinburgh (ed., *Report of Proc.*, Scottish Society of the History of Medicine) for information on Scottish developments. See also Rosemary Stevens, *Medical Practice in Modern England* (New Haven: 1966), pp. 24 f.

much to advance both basic and applied fields. Back of this contrast, apparently, there lurked a basic divergence in attitudes. Liebig summed this up in 1844 in the remark that in Britain [as also in the U.S.A] "only those works which have a practical tendency awake attention and command respect . . . In Germany it is quite the contrary."[60]

The implications of this contrast for medical teaching and research prior to 1890 are in retrospect obvious enough. It may be added however, that the direct influence exerted by these attitudes often took financial form. This is well brought out in an account, said to have been given by Macaulay in his diary for January 14, 1851, of a conversation held with Prince Albert:

> I remarked [Macaulay stated] that it was impossible to make either Oxford or Cambridge a great medical school. He said, truly enough, that Oxford and Cambridge are larger towns than Heidelberg, and yet that Heidelberg is eminent as a place of medical education. He added . . . why this was. There was hardly, he said, a physician in Germany . . . who made one thousand pounds a year by his profession. In that case, a professorship at Heidelberg may well be worth as much as the best practice in the great cities. Here, where Brodie and Bright make more than ten thousand pounds a year, and where, if settled at Cambridge or Oxford, they probably could not make fifteen hundred pounds, there is no chance that the academic chairs will be filled by the heads of the profession.

Brodie and Bright could, of course, teach in London, though even there successful practice inhibited original studies among members of the medical faculties.[61]

It is not surprising, therefore, that even when German-type research invaded "Oxbridge," the universities continued to send medical students to London for clinical training. And in the

[60] D. S. L. Cardwell, *The Organization of Science in England* (London: Heinemann, 1957), pp. 49–51. See also George Haines, IV, *German Influence upon English Education and Science* (New London: 1957), especially chap. 4.

[61] Newman, *Evolution of Medical Education* (n. 16, above), chap. 6; R. H. Shryock, *American Medical Research* (New York: Commonwealth Fund, 1947), pp. 30–32, 68–72. The quotation from Macaulay is given in O. H. Wangensteen, "Then and Now—The Surgical Arena Three Decades Ago," *Jour. Lancet* (Minneapolis), vol. 77 (November, 1957), pp. 401 f.

schools there, traditional professors—the great practitioners—avoided specialization and research much as did their counterparts in Philadelphia or Boston. One can understand their attitude but it involved rear guard action at best. By 1900 or 1910 a new generation was trying to reconcile, if not actually to blend, basic research and clinical studies in both the London and the provincial faculties.

In consequence, the goal of more than fifty years of reform—the "safe general practitioner"—began to emerge from improved schools and to pass examinations which approached uniformity in scope and quality. Only vestiges of distinct grades of doctors survived in the prestige of licentiates of the Conjoint Board in England, and in the emergence of qualifications for surgeons and consultants not required of other practitioners.

Parenthetically, examinations were improved by a shift from oral quizzes to more searching, written tests which came into use after 1850. This trend was both cause and effect of rising standards. ("Orals" had been insulated from outside criticism.) Here was an early instance of advancement in testing—a field which held promise for the future in medicine as well as in other fields.[62]

It required another decade or two before the educational phase of this achievement was attained in the United States, and a still longer interval before examining procedures would become even more centralized than those established in Britain. In order to follow this story one must return again to the transatlantic scene at mid-century, that is, to a time when medical reform was being advocated as urgently in America as it was in western Europe.

[62] Carr-Saunders, *The Professions* (n. 3, above), p. 310; F. Beach, "On Recent Legislation in Relation to the Medical Profession," *British Med. Jour.,* 1 (1900), pp. 371–73. On the provincial schools which began to be established in the 1820s, see, e.g. E. M. Brockband, *The Foundation of Provincial Medical Education in England, and of the Manchester School in Particular* (Manchester: Manchester Univ. Press, 1936), *passim.*

CHAPTER II † MEDICAL REFORM: ACHIEVEMENTS AND LIMITATIONS, 1875–1965

Professional leaders in "the States" were by no means ignorant of British trends, and they became equally aware of German institutions after 1870. Prior to the Civil War there had been some ridicule—especially in the Middle West—of subservience to European medicine,[63] but this was silenced by the growing promise in such fields as bacteriology and biochemistry. For some years, nevertheless, American doctors were slower than those in Britain in reacting to Teutonic progress. Upon returning from abroad they saw little hope of reforming their schools in the German image. William H. Welch declared in 1878 that the state of native medical education was "simply horrible."[64]

Despite democratic strivings, resistance to reform was still encouraged by the assumption that second-grade doctors could care for the poor. Reassuring, in any case, was the old view that innate talents might make up for the lack of formal instruction. "It may be said," Dr. James McNaughton of the Albany Medical College had declared in 1847,

> that the lives of the poor . . . are as valuable as those of the rich, and that, therefore, they ought to have as good physicians and surgeons . . . but we must take the world as we find it. In every country the great mass . . . are attended by medical men of inferior acquirements [yet] it often happens that the comparatively illiterate general practitioner is a better and safer medical advisor than the graduated and finished scholar.[65]

[63] T. N. Bonner, *American Doctors and German Universities* . . . (Lincoln: Univ. of Nebraska Press, 1963), pp. 8 f.

[64] James and Simon Flexner, *William H. Welch* . . . (New York: Viking, 1941), p. 113. See also J. Ben-David, "Scientific Productivity and Academic Organization in the Nineteenth Century," *Amer. Sociol. Rev.,* vol. 25 (December, 1960), pp. 828 ff.

[65] *Proc. of the National Medical Conventions* (Philadelphia: 1847), pp. 111 f. The final statement here was an expression of the view mentioned in n. 8, above.

Note, however, that even in this statement Dr. McNaughton recognized a dawning desire for first-rate medicine for all the people.

Such sentiment increased with the impact of German science, since this accentuated contrasts between the old practice and the new. Exciting vistas in surgery, preventive medicine, and pharmacology—all revealed by "regular" medicine—were impressing the public by the 1880s. True, something of the clinical nihilism inherited from Paris and Vienna persisted until the end of the century. This was just as well for the time being. Promiscuous bleeding and purging declined after 1850 and were vestigial by the 1870s,[66] and in the meantime such dramatic achievements as those of Pasteur, Koch, and Lister no longer could be ignored.

Homeopaths and eclectics, whose origins went back to the learned medicine of an earlier day, were impressed and began to blend their teachings with those of the new allopathy. Public cynicism gradually declined, and the sectarian crusade for medical freedom lost much of its earlier vigor. New sects did appear, but one—so-called Christian Science—was a form of religious healing; while osteopathy, at first a doctrinaire cult, flourished over the years only by following homeopathy back along the road toward regular medicine.[67]

[66] For a belated defense of bloodletting, see the *Arnold Letters* (n. 50, above), pp. 135 ff. (1868). But by 1886 the distinguished Dr. Austin Flint of New York was urging that the procedure be used only with great discretion—as it still is on occasion; see his *Medicine of the Future* (New York: 1886), an address prepared for the British Medical Association. An analysis of the whole trend is provided by L. S. Bryan, Jr., "Blood Letting in American Medicine, 1830–1892," *Bull. of the Hist. of Med.*, vol. 38 (1964), pp. 516–29.

[67] Homeopathy became almost indistinguishable from regular medicine after 1920, and in recent decades osteopathy has been moving in the same direction. I know of no critical study of just how this latter metamorphosis has been accomplished. On osteopathy, see A. T. Still, *Autobiography* (Kirkville, Mo.: 1897), *passim;* and for a sympathetic account of all the sects, A. Wilder, *History of Medicine . . .* (New Sharon, Me.: 1901), pp. 416–40, 776–835. Note also R. P. Keesecker, ed., *The Osteopathic Movement in Medicine: A Source Document . . . (1892–1957)* (Chicago: Amer. Osteo. Assoc., 1957), 24 pp., bibliog.; D. B. Thorburn, "The Case for Osteopathy," *Amer. Mercury*, LXX (January, 1950), 32–42; and J. D. Wassersug, "The Medical Position— A Reply," *ibid.*, pp. 42–50.

Thus, without fully anticipating it, medical reformers entered an era after 1850 when several factors converged to promote their cause. One can observe among them during the 1850s both disillusionment and continued hope for the future. When degrees were so discredited by poor schools it had been proposed that medical societies should again take over control of licensing. It was suggested, for example, that membership in the national society would provide better certification than the possession of a degree. Such letters as M.A.M.A. (member, American Medical Association) might prove superior to an M.D. When the association itself did not encourage this idea, the better faculties made intermittent attempts to raise their own standards from within.

In other words, efforts to improve education and licensing were never entirely given up despite the failures of the A.M.A. Although the University of Pennsylvania abandoned in 1853 a term lengthened to six months because other schools declined to follow, the Penn Medical University (eclectic) announced "progressive (graded) courses" within the next year. Five years later a Chicago college (later Northwestern University) introduced a three-year, graded curriculum with six-month terms and annual tests in each subject. The Civil War doubtless delayed further experiment, and for several decades after 1865 the A.M.A. made little effort to improve matters. Progressive doctors then by-passed it by arranging informal conventions to urge innovations similar to those adopted at Northwestern. Such meetings were held at Cincinnati in 1867, at Washington, D.C. in 1870 and at Chicago in 1876, and all placed emphasis upon graded programs and annual, written examinations of each class.

Several schools finally began to move with the times during the 1870s. At Harvard a research laboratory in physiology was established in 1871, the academic year was increased to nine months, and a graded curriculum and regular examinations were provided. The immediate result was a decline in enrollments, to offset which the university provided salaries in the place of student fees. Several other schools had followed this example by 1876. Pennsylvania, which adopted similar arrangements in 1877, had three years before provided another innovation of basic value. This was the founding, under Provost Pepper, of its own University Hospital which assured faculty control of clinical teaching. Several other schools soon made the same arrangement or strengthened connections with hospitals, so that such teaching—though still a passive experience for most students—became the rule in these colleges. It was this clinical program, superior in most respects to the old single-preceptor relationship, which led to the abandonment of apprenticeships during the 1870s and 1880s.

As long as entrance requirements had involved little more than apprenticeship few improvements could be made because there was no control over the hundreds of preceptors, but as soon as students came directly from high schools (secondary schools) to the medical colleges academic prerequisites could be demanded. No doubt some price was paid for this achievement, since the students were no longer introduced early to the realities of practice. In French schools even first-year students were taken into the hospitals, but as graded, lengthened curricula developed in America, clinical training was put off until the third or fourth years. This arrangement, of course, had its own merits, but it may be noted, looking ahead, that after World War II several schools set up programs—chiefly in "family practice"—in an attempt to recover values once attributed to apprenticeships.

Such advances as those noted were still limited during the 1870s to a few of the most progressive schools. But they did represent some response to German influences. Between 1875 and 1914 about fifteen thousand American doctors returned from abroad with an awareness of real clinical teaching; of close relations between hospitals and schools; of specialization and full-time, salaried professorships; and above all, of the possibility of transforming both teaching and practice through close association with research. Such men were a small minority in the American profession before 1900, but they were beginning to be heard in the major centers.

Thus N. S. Davis of Chicago, in his A.M.A. presidential address of 1883, announced that educational reform now demanded (1) premedical, academic requirements; (2) minimal time in medical-school and hospital training; (3) state boards to provide licensing examinations; and (4) the strengthening of professional societies to attain these ends. Here was a program for medical reform envisaged by a founder of the A.M.A. still optimistic after more than thirty-five years of seeming futility. Only in regard to specialization which Davis (and many others) viewed as a threat to guild solidarity, did he oppose the latest professional trends.[68]

Dr. Davis did not advocate a return to licensing by state societies, but he hoped that these bodies could persuade legislatures to place control in the hands of the states. The vital point was to take this power away from the schools. Even opposition expressed against parts of his program pointed in the same direction. For example, critics held that it made no difference whether a year was added to courses, *provided* graduates must in any case pass state examinations. If a man could become a competent physician after only two years of study, why make him spend three years in a medical college?

It was no coincidence, then, that an era of educational reform witnessed the revival of direct licensing by state boards. Even

[68] See the *Medical and Surgical Reporter,* n.s., I (1859), 283, *re* the letters "M.A.M.A." On early educational reforms, note Corner, *Two Centuries of Medicine* (n. 29, above), pp. 126, 133–42; Davis, *Medical Education and Medical Institutions* (n. 38, above), pp. 48 f.; the *Jour. of the Amer. Med. Assoc.,* I (1883), 33–42; Shryock, *Medical Research* (n. 61, above), chap. 2; and H. J. Abrahams, "Extinct Medical Schools of Philadelphia: (VIII) Summary and Conclusions," *Trans.* College of Physicians of Philadelphia, 4 ser., vol. 32 (July, 1964), p. 41.

states which had never before provided controls now began to do so. Kentucky, for example, authorized the governor in 1874 to appoint five doctors in each judicial district as examiners. More common, when tests were imposed for the first time, was the provision of a single examining board. There were exceptions: two eastern and a number of states west of the Mississippi did not establish examining systems until the present century. Practically all states which had maintained boards prior to 1850, however, re-established them before 1900.

Events within any single state, however, were often frustrating to the medical societies concerned. As an illustration, in the case of the states hitherto lacking controls, one may select Pennsylvania. In this prosperous commonwealth efforts to secure a licensing body were rebuffed for more than a century. Abandoning hope for official regulations, some 125 Philadelphia doctors had tried in 1877 to form an unofficial examining body. Their scheme, which reminds one of Dr. Morgan's efforts a century earlier, met a similar fate—the state refused to charter a voluntary board at the same time that it failed to provide one of its own.

In 1881 the Legislature did set up a registration system. This lacked the legal aspects of the British Register but may have served to identify respectable men. Parenthetically, the Pennsylvania Register now throws light on the distribution of personnel in a large community. In Philadelphia in 1881, some 1,480 doctors ministered to a population of 850,000: a typical American ratio of about 1:570. Among the total, 237 were homeopaths and 49 were women—all but 7 of the latter, graduates of the Woman's Medical College in that city. Not until 1893 did Pennsylvania, long a center of medical education, finally establish a state examining board.[69]

[69] On Kentucky, see K. W. Rawlings, ed., *Medicine and Its Development in Kentucky* (Louisville: 1940), p. 263; on Pennsylvania, *The Physician's Protective Register* (Philadelphia: 1881), *passim;* H. F. Alderfer, "Legislative History of Medical Licensure in Pennsylvania," *Penna. Med. Jour.,* vol. 64

Among states which revived earlier controls, one of the most interesting cases was that of Louisiana. Severe requirements had been provided there as early as 1723, because the French— like the Spanish—attempted an immediate projection of medical codes overseas. (Violations of the first New Orleans regulations had been, in theory, punishable by death!) After American annexation in 1804, New Orleans had set up a board which tested even men holding M.D. degrees—perhaps the only instance of such a policy as late as 1820. Later acts weakened French requirements, however, and testing was abandoned in 1852 in accordance with the prevailing trend. In the 1870s the state medical society revived a demand for effective licensure, and finally an Act of 1894 provided that two state boards should examine all candidates. Not until 1908, however, were real penalties attached for non-compliance.

Several later Louisiana measures included provisions not uncommon during this second stage of legislation—1875 to 1900. Midwives as well as pharmacists in New Orleans were examined by the state boards, and men holding "satisfactory" licenses from other states or from foreign countries were admitted to practice without reference to reciprocity.[70]

Rural midwives, however, were not examined. Their practice was largely among Negroes, and here one observes a formal vestige of low-grade service for low-income families. Such neglect was typical of most southern states for decades thereafter and constituted the most blatant weakness in American practice after 1920. The training and certification of mid-

---

(1961), pp. 1605–49. *Re* objections to longer courses, see Y. H. Bond, "A Knowledge or a Time Requirement . . .?", *Jour. of the Amer. Med. Assoc.* (May 2, 1891), pp. 625 f., who claimed that in 1890 about 40 per cent of German graduates—after long courses—failed the state medical examinations.

[70] John Duffy, in organizing and writing *The Rudolph Matas History of Medicine in Louisiana* (Baton Rouge: Louisiana State Univ. Press, 1958, 1961), provides one of the most detailed accounts of any state's history of licensure; see vol. I, chap. 15, and vol. II, chap. 15. Articles have appeared on various other states, e.g., L. G. Caldwell, "Early Legislation Regulating the Practice of Medicine," *Illinois Law Rev.,* vol. 18 (December, 1923), pp. 242–44, *re* Illinois.

wives was casual even in northern states, where their services were desired chiefly by immigrant families. The situation reflected an apparently class-conscious indifference to such practice, for it persisted even after European countries improved training and testing in this specialty. As late as 1900 some twenty states provided no controls whatever.

Thereafter, a few specialists in good schools demanded better teaching of obstetrics and the elimination of "dirty and ignorant" midwives. It was difficult to arouse the public, however, in view of the common opinion that birth was "just a natural process." And even though almost 50 per cent of all births were still reported by midwives as late as 1910, general practitioners were probably not too much concerned about competition for the patronage of the poor. Moreover, the actual record of the "G.P.s" in this field was sometimes inferior to that of the "granny women." Some reform in training and testing finally evolved, however, as obstetrical teaching improved, and as the immigrant population declined after 1920.[71]

The same society which often ignored midwives was also antagonistic to women as general practitioners. When the Woman's Medical College was founded in Philadelphia in 1850, reflecting the feminist movement, many laymen and most physicians condemned the program in violent terms. Resistance to this invasion of a man's world persisted longer in the United States than in some European countries, hence American women decided to organize additional schools open only to their sex.

[71] There is more historical literature on British than on American midwifery. On the former, note, e.g., J. H. Aveling, *English Midwives* (London: Churchill, 1872), *passim;* Carr-Saunders *The Professions* (n. 3, above) pp. 122–25; G. P. McClear, *The Maternity and Child Welfare Movement* (London; King and Son, 1935), pp. 131–70; and Jeanne A. Brand, *Doctors and the State* (Baltimore: The Johns Hopkins Press, 1965), pp. 178–80. A protest against the early decline of American midwifery is expressed in S. Gregory, *Man-Midwifery Exposed and Corrected* (Boston: 1848), pp. 18 ff.; and an analysis of further decline since 1900 is given in Frances E. Kobrin, "The American Midwife Controversy: A Crisis of Professionalization," *Bull. of the Hist. of Med.,* XL (July–August, 1966), 350–63.

At this point their limited success was made possible by the very weaknesses in education and licensing which were otherwise so deplorable. In the first place, legislatures which gave charters to any doctors who wished to found a school could be persuaded to oblige a few men willing to educate women. In the second place, though these "female colleges" were struggling institutions their graduates—whether well trained or not —were sure to be licensed if granted degrees.

Prior to the 1890s no major American schools admitted women (Swiss universities opened their doors in the 1870s), but this could not prevent "the doctoring ladies" from qualifying for practice. They were further aided by considerable newspaper support and by a liberal attitude in some sectarian colleges. Even so, women were excluded from medical societies and hospitals for two decades or more, while the members of these bodies ostracized them professionally even as they did irregulars. By the 1890s western state universities began to admit women to their medical colleges, but most of the better eastern institutions did so only between 1900 and 1940.[72] One well-known school excluded them until the 1960s.

Somewhat similar treatment was accorded Negro physicians when a medical school was set up in Howard University—an institution founded for that race by the federal government soon after the Civil War. Denied admittance to the A.M.A., Negro doctors finally organized their own National Medical Association in 1870.[73]

It seems ironic, in view of the disdain expressed for sectarians, that "regulars" in most states finally secured regulations only

[72] R. H. Shryock, "Women in American Medicine," *Jour. of the Amer. Med. Women's Assoc.,* V (September, 1950), 371–79. For earlier recognition in Europe, see J. Steudel, "Heilkundige Frauen des Abendlandes," *Zentralblatt für Gynäkologie,* Heft 8 (1959), pp. 284 ff.

[73] E. E. Konold, *A History of American Medical Ethics, 1847–1912* (Madison: State Hist. Soc. of Wis., 1962), p. 24; W. M. Cobb, *The First Negro Medical Society* (Washington, D.C.: Associated Publishers, 1939), chaps. I–IV, incl. Cf. D. C. Reitzes, *Negroes and Medicine* (Cambridge: Harvard Univ. Press, 1958), for recent trends.

with the aid of homeopaths and/or eclectics. Cooperation was encouraged not only by political realism but also by the convergence of forms of practice which made such realism more palatable. As early as the mid-1870s both the Louisiana and the Michigan state societies agreed with homeopaths on setting up joint licensing boards, and Massachusetts in 1884 included eclectics in a single examining system. Tennessee, in founding its first board in 1889, included both homeopaths and eclectics among the members.[74] In some cases, however separate boards were provided for sectarians as well as for dentists and, eventually, for ancillary (paramedical) personnel. Certain legislatures even supported both homeopathic and regular schools within a single state university—as was the case in Ohio as late as the 1920s.

In a few instances, licensing powers were vested in state boards of health. Between 1790 and 1860 local health offices had been set up in nearly all large cities, and cumulative efforts by these bodies and some medical societies led to the founding of twenty state boards between 1870 and 1880. Moreover, after national sanitary conventions had been halted by the Civil War, doctors joined with government officials in 1872 to form the American Public Health Association. Some of the medical men involved, disillusioned about the A.M.A., hoped that the new A.P.H.A. might take over the former's educational goals. Thus, Dr. Richard Arnold of Savannah (who had been the first secretary of the national medical society) wrote in 1872: "I have long considered it [the A.M.A.] a failure in regard to the advancement of medical science or medical education," but then added that he had high hopes for the A.P.H.A.

By the 1880s, moreover, the role of public health agencies was expanded by the impact of bacteriology on public hygiene. Up to this time, demographers and engineers had provided

---

[74] Konold, *American Medical Ethics* (n. 73, above), p. 27; Hamer, *Tennessee State Medical Association* (n. 47, above), p. 101.

much of the leadership in sanitation programs, but thereafter a small but able group of physicians took over. These men were public-spirited and professionally competent, and it is not strange that certain states utilized them as licensing authorities.[75]

Outstanding in this context was the Illinois Board of Health. This body, founded in 1877, was given authority to keep a list of recognized doctors. Men already in practice were directed to register their diplomas with the board for approval, and it is interesting that many of the older physicians absolutely refused to do this—viewing the requirement as an entering wedge to state medicine. The board persevered, however, and raised its sights to include medical schools outside the state. In 1880 it prepared a schedule of such schools "in good standing"— presumably for guidance in accepting degrees presented by candidates for licensure. Between 1883 and 1889, the board issued five formal reports in which it observed progress in the direction urged by presidents of the A.M.A., that is, toward extension of course terms and of total time in medical schools. The same trend was noted and approved by national societies of homeopathic and of eclectic practitioners.

Whether or not the Illinois board originally envisaged the function, it was soon engaged in reporting on all medical colleges in the United States and in Canada. Its criteria for approval were similar to those of N. S. Davis. Good schools should require (1) moral character, (2) pre-medical education through high school, (3) a curriculum including at least ten subjects, (4) two courses in dissection and two terms of hospital instruction, and (5) at least three years of training all told—although time spent with a preceptor could still be counted toward this total. Most meticulous, finally, were cer-

[75] R. H. Shryock, "Letters of R. D. Arnold . . .," Pt. II, *Bull. of the Johns Hopkins Hosp.*, XLII (April, 1928), 238; also *Medicine and Society* (n. 29, above), pp. 102 f., 163–65; and *The Development of Modern Medicine* (New York: Knopf, 1947), pp. 234 f., 239–41.

tain pedagogical requirements; regular attendance, at least two quizzes per week, and final examinations given preferably by men from outside the faculty. The annual reports included data on a great number of colleges, real or otherwise. That for 1889, for example, analyzed no less than 179 regular schools (16 in Canada), 26 homeopathic, 26 eclectic, 13 of other sects, and 13 indicted as "fraudulent."

The board's data may have been drawn simply from catalogues, yet its publications attracted attention in newspapers as well as in medical journals. Speaking in 1894, Dr. W. W. Keen —a well-known Philadelphia surgeon—stated that reform in medical education was first promoted by "the noble Illinois State Board of Health" which finally set "an advanced standard." The reports of this agency may have exerted more influence during the 1880s than did reforms in any particular college. At any rate, the idea of grading schools—however tentative—was implicit in the board's criteria; and within another decade this idea would be formally implemented by the A.M.A.[76]

Dr. Keen added that, although health boards now existed in nearly all states their work had been followed by "the still more notable advance of boards of medical examiners." He may have meant that, in licensing, such health agencies as had been active had been superseded by independent boards. Not many health offices had actually served as licensing bodies, and those which did soon found their hands full with new programs in public hygiene. Meantime, separate examining boards continued to be set up during the 1880s and 1890s, and by 1898

---

[76] *Report on Medical Education and the Regulation of the Practice of Medicine in the U.S. and Canada* (Springfield: Ill. State Board of Health, 1883); and similar *Report* for 1889, *passim*. Keen's remarks appear in his *Addresses and Other Papers* (Philadelphia: Saunders, 1905), pp. 195 ff. See also Bonner, *Medicine in Chicago* (n. 50, above), pp. 112, 114, who notes that even the Illinois board later ceased to exert any real control; and Black, "Medical Practitioners" (n. 139, below), *re* attitudes of older Illinois doctors toward the board.

only the Alaska Territory had no regulations whatever. In Michigan and five states west of the Mississippi the registration of any diploma entitled a man to practice, and eleven states still accepted either approved diplomas or examinations. But there were already twenty-two states which required both diplomas and state examinations—the program of the future.[77]

Most state boards were thus moving toward better standards (1875–1900), but this trend reflected more than new attitudes in official agencies. As early as 1876 progressive faculties had founded the Association of American Medical Colleges in order to promote reform from within. Although twenty-two colleges were represented at the first meeting, this effort was premature and was abandoned in 1883. (It was in that year that the Illinois Board of Health assumed leadership in judging diplomas.) Seven years later, after the board had issued its reports, medical faculties reasserted themselves by reviving the association. At the call of colleges in Baltimore and of the staff of the Johns Hopkins Hospital (opened in 1889), some sixty-five regular schools sent representatives to a meeting in Nashville. Nathan Smith Davis was again elected president (he had held the same office in 1879) and served until 1894. The association immediately called for a three-year curriculum, and grew during ensuing decades into a representative and influential body.[78]

Cumulative efforts to improve licensing soon led state examiners to organize on their own behalf. In 1891 they founded the National Confederation of State Medical Examining and Licensing Boards, which enabled them to exchange ideas and to plan more strict requirements. The boards, influenced by the better faculties, became aware of the leverage they in turn could exert on inferior schools. In 1891 the confederation

---

[77] W. R. Fisher, "Legal Restriction of Medical Practice," *Arena,* vol. 19 (1898), pp. 527–34.

[78] D. F. Smiley, "History of the Association of American Medical Colleges," *Jour. Med. Educ.,* vol. 32 (1957), pp. 512–18.

agreed with the Association of Medical Colleges in recommending three-year courses; in 1896 it urged that graduation from high school be made a minimum entrance requirement; and in 1904 it adopted a uniform curriculum recommended to all faculties.[79]

Meantime, the medical profession was given further impetus toward reform by the founding of scientific societies and of groups of specialists. Among the first type were the Association of American Physicians (1885) and the American Academy of Medicine (1890). A few organizations of specialists had appeared early—i.e., the New York Pathological Society (1844), the American Otological Society (1869), and the American Surgical Association (1880)—but their number increased rapidly thereafter, as in the founding of the Physiological Society in 1887, of the Pediatric Society in 1888, and of other surgical bodies between 1886 and 1913, culminating in the latter year in the establishment of the American College of Surgeons. Many members of these societies were at first only part-time specialists, but as they gradually gave more heed to one type of practice they became aware of the need for improved training in that field.[80]

As more groups outside the American Medical Association called for reform signs of change began to appear within that conservative body. The *Journal* was founded in 1883 (replacing the old *Transactions*), and an unsuccessful effort to modernize the association was made in 1886. Four years later the *Journal* urged recognition for the research worker—a note that was significant even though it was some fifty years overdue.

[79] W. L. Bierring, "Medical Licensure after Forty Years," *Conn. State Med. Jour.,* vol. 20 (1956), pp. 724–29.

[80] See, e.g., *Bulletin of the National Research Council,* no. 101 (October, 1937); and R. S. Bates, *Scientific Societies in the United States* (New York: John Wiley, 1945), p. 85; J. H. Means, *The Association of American Physicians: Its First Seventy-Five Years* (New York: McGraw-Hill, 1961), chaps. 1–3, incl.

Finally, in 1901, a general reorganization was adopted on the present federal basis. More able leadership and structural flexibility came in with the new dispensation.[81]

These developments, although initiated by trends within medicine (i.e., the German research drive and its achievements), also reflected changes within the social environment. The implications of urbanization, increasing wealth, and business efficiency were not lost on leading physicians. Competing within a free economy they observed that the scientific motive for educational reform coincided with their own professional ambitions. They became increasingly aware that too many schools were turning out too many graduates to make practice profitable.[82] This does not imply that educational and scientific appeals were mere hypocrisy. It simply means that these were so intertwined with economic interests as to make conclusions about the relative potency of each motivation almost impossible.

Another social factor encouraging reform was the growing concentration of wealth in the hands of business leaders. A few of the newly-made millionaires became major philanthropists, and several of the latter—like the well-educated public at large—were impressed by the possibilities of the new medicine. Mr. Johns Hopkins founded in Baltimore the first real university in the United States in 1876, and his bequest endowed a modern hospital there in 1889. In 1893 this hospital was coordinated with a new medical school patterned after its German prototype. For several decades thereafter "The Hopkins"—more than any other single institution—became the model for medical reform. From the start it required an arts degree for admission, provided a four-year graded course,

---

[81] Burrow, *AMA: Voice of American Medicine* (n. 48, above), pp. 33 ff.

[82] Complaints about low income had been common throughout the nineteenth century; see, e.g., T. Minor, *Annual Address . . . in the Medical Institution of Yale College* (New Haven: Hamlen, 1839), p. 3. But the attack on superfluous schools became more pronounced in this connection late in the century.

placed preclinical professors on a full-time basis, and emphasized freedom in both teaching and research.[83]

In the Baltimore school as elsewhere, however, all clinical teachers continued private practice. Unlike their German mentors, who as professors became rather insulated from practitioners, even the best American faculties were active in the medical societies. They led in the reorganization of the A.M.A. and thereafter urged it to support professional reform. After several years of such agitation, the association began to move more rapidly. In 1904 the *Journal* indicted even "regular" colleges as inferior, and stated that their number had grown from 90 in 1880 to 154—enough to supply the country with twice as many doctors as were needed to maintain already "absurdly crowded conditions." In the same year the association set up a Council on Medical Education, authorized to report annually to the House of Delegates on this whole subject. The Council held its first conference in 1905, where—in cooperation with representatives of licensing boards and of the Association of Medical Colleges—an "ideal standard" of education was adopted. This went beyond the one presented by the Illinois Health office in 1889, in that it called for the examination of all candidates by state boards.[84]

In the meantime, certain of these boards—adopting more strict requirements—refused to approve men licensed in other states. This trend involved new problems for graduates, and one way to ease the situation was for compatible boards to grant reciprocity in licensing. Such procedure was encouraged by correspondence between boards in the Middle West, and in 1902 a Confederation of Reciprocity was founded in Chicago. At that time, indeed, a few doctors looked beyond reciprocity. In 1903, for example, Dr. S. B. Lyon of Los Angeles urged

[83] Alan Chesney, *The Johns Hopkins Hospital and The Johns Hopkins University School of Medicine* (Baltimore: The Johns Hopkins Press, 1934), I, *passim*.

[84] Burrow, *AMA: Voice of American Medicine* (n. 48, above), pp. 33 ff.

that some voluntary body be formed to grant "a universal practitioner's license."[85] Perhaps he was aware of the concomitant appeal in Britain for a "single portal" to practice, but the idea must have seemed utopian to most Americans.

More realistic, in 1903, were the continued efforts of the Reciprocity Confederation to encourage inter-board agreements. After six years, however, this body included representatives from only about fifteen state agencies—nearly all of them west of the Appalachians. In 1912 it merged with the National Confederation of State Boards to form the present Federation of State Medical Boards.[86]

During the two decades 1890–1910, a considerable number of organizations were thus seeking to raise professional standards. The citadel of conservatism did not collapse immediately, however, despite all the trumpets proclaiming reform. The very urgency of these blasts suggests that there was still much resistance to overcome. Sectarians and cultists even undertook a counter-offensive. They viewed reformers as bigots who would suppress freedom in medical practice while upholding it in other spheres. Restrictions favoring "regulars" were termed reverberations from the seventeenth century.

During the 1890s a National Constitutional Liberty League was founded in Boston, which lobbied against strict requirements and distributed literature to the public. Those sympathetic to this cause could quote influential figures in support, notably English leaders (Gladstone and Huxley) who maintained the *caveat emptor* tradition. Even the American Samuel Clemens (Mark Twain)— who would later ridicule Christian Scientists—was said to have remarked:

> I don't know that I cared much about these osteopaths until I heard you were going to drive them out of the State; but since I heard this I haven't been able to sleep . . . . Now what I contend is that my body

<hr>

[85] Letter in the *Jour. of the Amer. Med. Assoc.* (October 10, 1903), p. 919.
[86] Bierring, *Medical Licensure* (n. 79, above), pp. 724–29.

59

is my own, at least I have always so regarded it. If I do harm through my experimenting with it, it is I who suffer, not the State.[87]

As late as 1901, Dr. A. Wilder (an eclectic) published a *History of Medicine* which presented a temperate defense of the sects.

During the decades 1890–1910, many inferior schools continued to flourish, and effective licensing regulations had not yet been provided in certain states. In 1898 Dr. L. Connor told the American Academy of Medicine that the profession still contained "a vast number of incompetents, large numbers of moral degenerates, crowds of pure tradesmen" and so on. In 1904 five states alone harbored fifty-four medical colleges, of which only six at best could be considered acceptable. And eleven years after The Hopkins required an arts degree for admission only five other schools insisted on *any* premedical education above the high school level. Some prominent physicians would later recall the mediocrity which persisted into this era. Thus Dr. Simon Flexner, first president of the Rockefeller Institute, remarked that at the two-year school from which he graduated about 1890: "I did not learn to practice medicine . . . indeed I cannot say that I was particularly helped by the school. What it did for me was to give me the M.D. degree."[88]

Despite such conditions, one can now see that the end of the century was a turning point in professional status. Although groups representing certain schools and boards had taken the initiative in reform before 1900, it was not until the A.M.A. was reorganized in 1901 that the full weight of the profession began to be exerted in this direction. As noted, the A.M.A. Council on Medical Education held its first conference in co-

[87] See Henry Wood, "Medical Slavery through Legislation," *Arena*, vol. 8 (1893), pp. 680–89; G. S. Andrews, "Medical Practice and the Law," *Forum*, vol. 31 (1901), p. 547.

[88] *Jour. of the Amer. Med. Assoc.*, vol. 32 (February 11, 1899), p. 273; Flexner autobiography, MSS, Amer. Phil. Soc. (Philadelphia).

operation with the state boards in 1904 and adopted an "ideal standard" of medical education.

Subsequently, the council also recommended full-time pre-clinical chairs, improved clinical training in hospitals (The Hopkins was already appointing third- and fourth-year students as "clinical clerks" or "surgical dressers"), and a search for endowments. Income from gifts could aid professors who no longer received student fees, and was essential to the extent that teaching and research became full-time functions and so were not supported by private practice. In recommending full-time preclinical chairs, the council was following Hopkins arrangements. But it may be anticipated here, that the council would not support that school when it extended full-time posts into clinical services in 1913. An intense controversy ensued over this issue. In the long run, full-time clinical appointments became more numerous though—with one exception—all schools retained many part-time clinical teachers.[89]

In effect, the A.M.A. council was saying by 1904 that if schools could not provide adequate education at a profit, they must give way to colleges supported by tuition, endowments and/or taxes. Such an outcome, combined with licensing controls, would put an end to schools which were proprietary in nature or inferior for other reasons. Similar trends could be observed in legal education, and one recalls that reform in both these professions coincided with public protests against the uncontrolled business domination of American society. Medical and political reformers were, in some degree, products of the same age.

After the A.M.A. council's second conference in 1906 it exposed inferior schools by publication of their graduates' records in state examinations—a more severe appraisal than

---

[89] D. Fleming, *William H. Welch* (Boston: Little, Brown, 1954), pp. 165–80; Shryock, *The Unique Influence of The Johns Hopkins University on American Medicine* (Copenhagen: Munksgaard, 1954), pp. 38–42.

anything attempted by the Illinois Board of Health in the 1880s. At a third conference in 1907 the council began to inspect and grade the schools, and as a result, thirty-two of these were rejected and forty-six more "conditioned." It was now clear that in the absence of federal legislation the voluntary association was at last returning to its original objective—the reform of the entire profession. In order to implement this program, a council committee made up of one hundred physicians recommended a survey of all the nation's medical schools.[90]

So ambitious a project was now feasible because of prospects for financial assistance. Several philanthropists had recently set up foundations so large as to permit aid to good works in general, rather than simply to a single program. Thus, Andrew Carnegie founded the institution named for him in Washington (1902), and John D. Rockefeller endowed the General Education Board (1903). The former in 1905, also established the Foundation for the Advancement of Teaching; and this body—under the direction of Henry S. Pritchett—undertook in 1909 the national survey desired by the A.M.A. council. Pritchett selected as director Abraham Flexner, a layman who combined ability and zeal with a knowledge of both European medical education and its American version at Hopkins.

Flexner then prepared the well-known study which was published by the foundation in 1910. He "pulled no punches" and revealed conditions no longer tolerable in the present century. "Bulletin Number Four" was dramatic, and perhaps exaggerated at some points, but its author and backers could not be accused—as a medical group might have been—of seeking selfish ends. The press took it up immediately and public opinion was aroused. State legislatures and licensing

---

[90] W. C. Rappleye, "Major Changes in Medical Education during the Past Fifty Years," *Jour. Med. Educ.*, vol. 34 (July, 1959), p. 684.

boards also responded and brought pressure to bear on medical schools to meet the standards laid down in the foundation report.

The outcome seemed miraculous to those not familiar with the efforts which had finally led up to the survey. All over the country, while the survey was under way as well as during the ensuing decade, medical schools closed, merged, or were reorganized along council lines. Proprietary colleges were abandoned, although income in private practice continued to benefit indirectly from faculty status, and independent (non-university) colleges were reduced to a few institutions in major cities. Meanwhile the A.M.A. Council on Medical Education developed its grading system on an A and B basis.

Most schools, between 1910 and 1930, began to insist on an arts degree for admission. This requirement may have raised standards, and the increasing maturity of students had advantages in itself. One may raise the question, nevertheless, whether a college education did not in part simply make up for a decline in the quality of secondary training? When the Illinois board had advocated graduation from high school as a premedical requirement in the 1880s, the few public high schools seem to have been select superior schools. So, likewise, were the better private academies. (One of the early public type still gives lawful bachelors' degrees.) Those trained in such schools may have been almost as well qualified academically in 1880 as were students who graduated both from the more popular high school and the average arts college of 1920.

By 1930 nearly all medical schools required an arts degree for admission and provided a three- or four-year, graded curriculum, improved hospital facilities, and clinical instruction. In addition, boards in some thirty states insisted—in cooperation with the American Hospital Association (founded in 1898) —that candidates take a year's internship as well as a recognized degree. The need for this supplementary clinical training became more obvious after the abandonment of apprenticeships.

As a result of these trends the ratings of medical colleges rose rapidly. In 1913, for example, twenty-four were graded A+, thirty-nine as A, and the rest as B. By 1918 out of the nearly sixty schools which were members of the Association of Medical Colleges fifty-six were graded A and only three listed as B. Although a number of low-grade schools still existed in that year, such colleges continued to disappear. A decade later the number of regular institutions had dropped to seventy-four and only five sectarian colleges survived, so that the total was about eighty—a remarkable decline from the 154 reported in 1904. (These figures do not include two-year, preclinical schools which passed students on into the third year of full-length programs.) By 1925 a B grade was rare, and during the 1930s and 1940s such a rating became a near catastrophe.

The decline in the number of schools slowed down after 1920, but continued until a low of sixty-six was reached in 1933. As anticipated, there was a consequent decline in the ratio of physicians from 1:600 in 1900 to about 1:763 by 1938. Thus the A.M.A., aided by certain foundations and supported by state boards, achieved both its goals by this decade; that is, an improvement in the selection and education of doctors, and a reduction in the ratio of doctors to population. The more careful selection of students was further encouraged by the growing prestige of medical science and a resulting improvement in the quality of men seeking medical education. Soon a wave of good students threatened to swamp the reduced number of schools. When the Duke college opened in 1932 only 68 applicants could be admitted though there were 3,000 inquiries.[91]

[91] Smiley, *Association of American Medical Colleges* (n. 78, above), p. 520; Shryock, *American Medical Research* (n. 61, above), pp. 119–21; Harris, *Economics of American Medicine* (n. 44, above), p. 111. On a superior high

Europeans had taken a dim view of American medicine during the nineteenth century. Such impressions had persisted until the 1890s, when foreign observers began reporting progress in the chief cities.[92] Dependence on German research and training declined thereafter and ended with World War I, after which the excellence of many schools in the United States was widely recognized. Yet few American physicians, despite their improving reputation, attempted to reverse the transit of culture by practicing in Europe. In this respect there was a sharp contrast with the achievements abroad of their colleagues in dentistry.

Occasionally, even before 1918, Americans had sought general practice in Britain, but they faced difficulties there because of ignorance of terminology and licensing codes. In 1891, for example, a certain S. E. L. Smith was registered in Birmingham as a licentiate of the Society of Apothecaries. He made the mistake, however, of announcing a degree and when taken into court produced a document describing himself as "M.D. Indianapolis." He was fined for claiming this degree, which the prosecutor declared was one of those American titles which could be secured for about thirty dollars.[93] It may have been just that.

In 1898, however, the indictment of another American revealed vestigial confusion in the British code itself. H. K. Hunter had taken a legitimate M.D. at Jefferson Medical College in Philadelphia, was a licentiate of the Society of Apothecaries (L.S.A.), and was practicing in Cambridgeshire. In all innocence, presumably because the two titles had long been interchangeable in the United States, he called himself "physician and surgeon." For this he was prosecuted by the General

school, see F. S. Edmonds, *History of the Central High School of Philadelphia* (Philadelphia: Lippincott, 1902) ; W. H. Cornog, *School of the Republic, 1893–1943* (Philadelphia: Assoc. Alumni, C.H.S., 1952). For the figures on Duke University I am indebted to the retired Dean, Dr. W. C. Davison.

[92] Bonner, *American Doctors and German Universities* (n. 63, above), chap. 5.

[93] *Jour. of the Amer. Med. Assoc.* (June 13, 1891), p. 864.

Medical Council (G.M.C.), which held that these honors still could be conferred only by the old medical corporations. Dr. Hunter was convicted and fined £5. When the Society of Apothecaries appealed, a higher court heard a prosecutor charge that although an L.S.A. was examined in both medicine and surgery he could not under the acts of 1815, 1858, and 1886, *term* himself a physician or surgeon. The defense denied this on the basis of the laws of 1858 and 1886. The judges, who had to search dictionaries for the connotation of "physician," upheld the prosecution in denying Dr. Hunter the use of these titles, but they agreed that he had not willfully misrepresented his status. The case was therefore dismissed, but Dr. Hunter had meanwhile died and so never learned of his vindication.

Throughout these hearings leading British physicians opposed the council's actions. Unlike the prosecution lawyers, they realized that old guild distinctions were now obsolete. As one observer put it:

> When the minds of all medical reformers have long been made up as to the desirability of securing . . . uniformity of qualification . . . it surely savours of retrogression for the G.M.C. to revive those distinctions which marked the intercollegiate jealousies of former days.

Or, as the neurologist Sir Victor Horsley remarked: the view of the prosecutor that the G.M.C. still divided the profession into three guilds was "wholly the outcome of an archaic imagination."[94] This case may have marked the last attempt to maintain guild lines in Britain, where "the safe general practitioner" was already coming on the scene. The date almost coincided with the reform of the A.M.A. in the United States, where certain schools were already turning out this same type of doctor.

During the years 1910–20, while American medical education was undergoing basic changes, licensing procedures were not

---

[94] *British Med. Jour.* (Jan. 28, 1899), pp. 225–27, 233–34; (Feb. 11, 1899), p. 375; (June 17, 1899), pp. 1484–85.

only made more strict but took on new and unexpected forms. In the first place, national societies of specialists began to scrutinize their own membership. Doctors who studied abroad became aware that it was not enough if a general practitioner specialized in one type of practice along with all his other work. Advanced (post-internship) clinical training was therefore introduced at The Hopkins in the 1890s, in the form of hospital "residencies" which were analogous to fellowships already provided in preclinical fields.[95]

Residencies were more complicated than most graduate education in that wards as well as laboratories and libraries were involved. The arrangement involved cooperation between a department and a teaching hospital and set up within the latter a special type of post-doctoral instruction. Hence it was not easy to adopt this program at once in all schools, nor could general practitioners be stopped from competing for the rewards of specialization. Some generalists would emphasize a particular type of practice, even though they were simply self-trained for this role or had assumed it by becoming an assistant to an established specialist. The latter device revived apprenticeship in a camouflaged form and had both the merits and limitations of that procedure. Another short-cut was to serve a specialized internship, but here also the amount of real instruction received was uncertain.[96]

The superiority of residency training was so obvious, however, that other medical schools introduced it during the years between about 1900 and 1920. The first to do so were those most concerned with research and resulting specialization, and those who were in a position to control hospital arrangements. The impact of The Hopkins' program was apparent in such

[95] Shryock, *American Medical Research* (n. 61, above), pp. 24–26; H. E. Sigerist, *American Medicine* (n. 8, above), p. 173.

[96] L. Davis, *Fellowship of Surgeons: A History of the American College of Surgeons* (Springfield, Ill.: Thomas, 1960), pp. 338–40.

cases, but some well-known schools not so influenced adopted residencies only after 1925.[97]

Even before this program was generally accepted, specialists' organizations sought to raise standards for admission, and the completion of an approved residency became the usual requirement. The question also arose: Should not the public be protected by some procedure—in effect, by additional licensing requirements—from doctors who claimed to be specialists? The state examining boards declined to become involved in this problem, and to this day the general license entitles the holder to pursue any type of practice. Whether the motive of the boards was just to avoid another responsibility, or whether it arose from the traditional antipathy to guild distinctions, is an academic question. Or it may be that specialists themselves preferred to keep controls out of official hands. In any case, the lack of government measures once more consigned a problem to voluntary professional bodies.

The first national society to rise to the occasion was that of the ophthalmologists, who in 1916 established a national board to certify doctors in this field. By 1945 no less than fourteen organizations of specialists had set up similar boards for their respective areas. These agencies continued to raise standards— much as had the general state boards before them—by providing examinations as well as by requiring approved education.[98]

In the case of surgical specialties, encouragement was provided by the American College of Surgeons (A.C.S.)—an élite body founded in 1913—which took over leadership in some degree from the American Surgical Association (1880). The college encountered opposition at first, on grounds that remind one of the objections to Dr. Morgan's plan for a col-

---

[97] See, e.g., Corner, *Two Centuries of Medicine* (n. 29, above) p. 278; Shryock, *American Medical Research* (n. 61, above), p. 26.

[98] B. J. Stern, *American Medical Practice* (New York: Commonwealth Fund, 1945), pp. 47–49.

lege of physicians during colonial days. The founders were accused of setting up a "Royal College" modeled on the old London corporations. But the persistent American view that democracy must be equated with mediocrity could not entirely hide the need for protecting the public. Such need was especially dramatic in the case of surgery. As Dr. Loyal Davis put it:

> Patients, with intelligent judgment in other matters, were cheerfully hopping up on operating tables and allowing a medical school graduate with one year of training in a rotating internship to . . . search aimlessly within their abdominal and other body cavities.[99]

Dr. Franklin Martin, founder of the A.C.S., had indeed been influenced by the British and Irish royal colleges and had also envisaged a supplementary specialists' degree as well as certification. The latter device was provided by all specialty boards, but the supplementary degree never took form.

The complexities involved in the evolution of some of these boards are again well illustrated in the case of surgery, wherein the American Surgical Association, the American College of Surgeons, specialty boards in such fields as gynecology and orthopedics, and the American Hospital Association all had to mesh their interests in the founding of the American Board of Surgery, in 1936.

The value of certification in a specialty—a sort of unofficial license—was soon recognized by well-informed doctors and by the better educated public.[100] Since there was no legal requirement for certification, however, many poor or less sophisticated families continued ·to be served entirely by general practitioners. It was said that more than half of all general surgery was still provided by men without specialized training.[101]

[99] Davis, *Fellowship of Surgeons* (n. 96, above), p. 444.

[100] *Ibid.*, pp. 89, 266, 439, 453. See also J. S. Rodman, *History of the American Board of Surgery* (Philadelphia: Lippincott, 1956), *passim.*

[101] Davis, *Fellowship of Surgeons* (n. 96, above), p. 444; E. R. Perez, "Challenge of the Future," *Bull. Amer. College of Surgeons,* vol. 38 (1953), p. 220; interview with Dr. I. S. Ravdin, *ibid.,* vol. 46, Pt. I, (1961), pp. 199–203; obituary Paul Hawley, *New York Times,* Nov. 26, 1965.

The education of specialists was only one of several problems with which state boards were unable or unwilling to cope. Although these bodies finally established standards for the basic license, most of them gave little heed to such issues as quackery, the need of older doctors for refresher training, and the confusion inherent in the existence of forty-eight independent jurisdictions. Each of these problems involved the quality of medical care as well as the interests of the profession, and so pertained to licensure in a broad sense of the term. Yet each was left for many years in the hands of voluntary medical organizations; indeed, only the suppression of quackery was finally attempted by official agencies. Even in the latter area the states were ineffective and it remained for the federal government to take over.

In contrast to British tradition, as noted, American state laws had at times condemned quackery. Late in the nineteenth century city authorities, prodded by political reformers, made sporadic attempts to enforce existing statutes. Thus, Theodore Roosevelt, when police commissioner of New York during the 1890s, tried to suppress "illicit practitioners."[102] During most of that century, however, quackery grew apace because of improved means for attracting victims. American versions of the ancient "medicine show" flourished, and testimonial techniques made a universal appeal. Charlatans, moreover, invented national advertising after cheap newspapers became available, and the patent-medicine evil soon became big business. Public apathy, suspicion that doctors wished to suppress competition, and the desperation of those beyond help also abetted quackery, but these had long been constant factors.

A bill to prohibit patent medicines had been introduced in Congress as early as 1849, but to no effect.[103] Similar indiffer-

[102] See the article by M. J. Lewis, in the *N. Y. State Jour. of Med.*, vol. 56 (1956), pp. 2135–36.

[103] *Congressional Globe*, March 3, 1849, p, 697; J. S. Billings, "American Invention and Discoveries in Medicine . . .," *Smithsonian Institution Annual Report* (1892), Pt. I (Washington: Gov't. Printing Office, 1893), p. 614.

ence was shown toward efforts to assure the reliability of drugs in general. A society which abandoned licensing could hardly be counted on to condemn any sort of practice, nor could much be expected from the American Medical Association until after that body was reorganized in 1901. One should remember, however, that there was a similarly lush growth of quackery in Europe during the same era.[104]

During the two decades following 1901, fortunately, revival of the A.M.A. coincided with social and political reforms of the "progressive era." Between 1900 and 1905 Upton Sinclair and other "muckrakers" exposed the food industries and aroused popular interest in food and drug legislation. Linked with this effort was the first real crusade against nostrums and patent medicine firms, which by 1900 numbered over 2,000 and each year produced materials valued at $60 million—about $300 million at today's prices. Here was a most irregular form of practice on a big-business scale. When Congress hesitated to move against any vested interest, the A.M.A. *Journal* published (in 1900) the first articles exposing proprietary remedies and promised also to remove quack advertising from its own pages.

This initial effort proved abortive, but in 1905 the association returned to the attack by forming its council on pharmacy and chemistry. The council examined both ethical and patent medicines, began the publication of *New and Nonofficial Remedies* (1907), and established contacts with liberal leaders in Congress and in the federal Department of Agriculture. After much lobbying in Congress that body finally passed the first food and drug act of 1906. This law proved ineffective, especially in relation to secret remedies, but in campaigning for it the A.M.A. established leadership in a continuing pressure on the federal government. In 1911 the association wired Presi-

---

[104] See, e.g., G. King, "Sale of Quack Medicines," *Provin. Med. and Surg. Jour.,* vol. 8 (1844), p. 596; R. R. Rentoul, "The Obligations of Medical Practitioners and Chemists . . . to the Public," *Med. Press and Circular,* n.s., vol. 52 (1892), p. 364; and statement in *Nature,* vol. 140 (October 16, 1937), pp. 660–61.

dent Taft that about 2,000,000 cases of illness and 500,000 deaths resulted annually from the use of impure food and drugs.

Pending opportunities to secure better legislation, the association set up its own chemical laboratory in 1906 and embarked on a program of direct exposure of fraudulent and dangerous remedies. In 1911 it published *Nostrums and Quackery,* which was well received. Also set up was a propaganda department to carry on the crusade. Meantime, the A.M.A. urged medical journals and even newspapers to drop all proprietary ads. It particularly denounced the cruelty of cancer and consumption "cures," and successfully defended itself against legal counter-measures taken by manufacturers. It later suppressed some of the most flamboyant individual quacks—e.g., the notorious John R. Brinkley, upon whom it conferred the title, "the greatest charlatan in medical history." Brinkley, like others, had ex-ploited the new mass medium of radio in the 1920s.

The fact remained that the Food and Drugs Act of 1906 was weak and set limits to what the embattled A.M.A. could accomplish. A renewed drive for federal legislation was there-fore launched in 1933, when the "New Deal" era once more provided a favorable opportunity. No effective laws were secured for several years, however, until the "sulfanilamide tragedy" of 1937 resulted in seventy-three deaths and dramatic-ally revealed the persisting lack of control of dangerous drugs. Congress reacted quickly in passing the Food, Drug, and Cos-metic Act of 1938, which required disclosure of contents on labels, imposed certain limitations on advertising, and banned new drugs before approval by a federal food and drugs ad-ministration. Although this act was not perfect and the A.M.A. decided that a national health department was needed to over-see the problem, the advent of some federal control had at last arrived.

During the next two decades the educated public felt reas-sured by the Act of 1938, and doubtless assumed that in an era of wonder-drugs the quacks would have little room to maneuver. But the resources of these mountebanks and the persistent credulity of their victims were underestimated. Charlatans found loopholes in even stringent legislation, and in 1957 the Postmaster General announced that the use of the mails to promote quackery was at the highest level in history. Even the old medicine show reappeared on television, camouflaged in the form of well-known entertainers who plugged their sponsor's product. Journalists, rediscovering quackery in electric gadgets, nutritional frauds, and the familiar cancer cures, declared that patent medicines were costing the public one billion dollars a year.

Cooperating with the A.M.A., however, the Food and Drug Administration (F.D.A.) and other federal agencies were now in a better position to suppress flagrant operators through court actions. In 1961 the F.D.A. and A.M.A. sponsored a National Congress on Medical Quackery, presumably to educate both Congress and the public. In any case, Congress passed during the next year a further law which greatly tightened requirements. This legislation is so strict that some pharmacologists even view it as too drastic: it now costs about $150,000 to introduce a single new drug on the market.[105]

One of the more subtle aspects of quackery was the extent to which licensed doctors themselves succumbed to its lures. But even more serious in lowering the quality of practice was the failure of medical men—particularly of general practitioners—to keep up with scientific innovations. This lag became

[105] Burrow, *AMA: Voice of American Medicine* (n. 48, above), chaps., 4, 6, and 13; G. Carson, *The Roguish World of Dr. Brinkley* (New York: Rinehart, 1960), *passim;* R. H. Shryock, *National Tuberculosis Association: 1904–1954* (New York: 1957), pp. 87 f. On present cost of introducing a new drug, see G. B. Koelle, in Annual Conference on Graduate Medical Education, *Proceeds.* ("Medicine in the Year 2000") (Philadelphia: 1964), p. 64. Cf. G. P. Larrick, "Appraising Drug Safety and Efficacy," *Emory Univ. Quarterly,* XXI (1965), 88–96. For information on quackery, 1938–62, I am indebted to a forthcoming article by Harvey Young, "Quackery, Incorporated."

more serious after 1890, and especially after 1930, as technical progress accelerated. Older physicians continued to give their patients service which was thirty years out of date. The problem confronted all professions but was most serious in medicine. Theoretically, the states might have required further training, additional tests, and renewed licenses every twenty years or so, but busy practitioners would have been overwhelmed by such requirements. In earlier periods the need to be brought up to date had been met by some doctors through sojourns abroad, but this custom declined with the improvements of American medical schools.

The first effort to meet the problem was the establishment in five or six cities of "postgraduate schools" which gave short courses for physicians, on an informal basis. In 1910 thirteen of these institutions were in operation. Thereafter, the development of residencies largely replaced such schools for a time. Gradually, however, the need for them reappeared as men wishing to specialize prepared for examinations. Medical veterans returning from World War II also sought "retreading" before taking up general practice again.

In 1946 a "Committee on Medicine in the Changing Order" of the New York Academy declared that: "Nothing would aid more in making medical practice adequate for great numbers of people than procedures by which these practitioners could keep in touch with advancing science." It added that association with a good hospital was the most immediate way to do this, but noted that many doctors lacked such connections.

Also advocated were refresher courses in medical centers. Experiments along this line had been tried here and there, as when the University of Michigan gave one-week courses twice a year, and granted a certificate—a sort of supplemental license—to men who completed 60 per cent of these courses over four years. By 1946 about a third of the state's doctors had been reached in this way. In other states, refreshing was limited to a few two- or three-day conferences each year. But at that time less than 25 per cent of the profession had availed itself of these opportunities.[106]

Efforts to provide in-residence, refresher training after World War II involved formal postgraduate schools in several universities, each with its own faculty and budget. In some cases, regular programs of two to nine months were provided—intended usually as preparation for specialty board examinations. More common were the refresher courses which ran anywhere from two days to two weeks, given usually by clinical departments within the schools. The constant difficulty, however, was the inability or unwillingness of doctors to leave their practice for any length of time, and for this reason courses given for only two or three days at local centers were usually best attended. The A.M.A. Council on Medical Education reported that in 1951–52, about 66,000 doctors received some sort of post graduate instruction. The common estimate still was, however, that less than 25 per cent of the profession was reached by these programs.[107]

It was urged that "group practice" would enable more doctors to secure refresher training, since individual members could be absent while the rest of the team carried on. Another claim for such practice was that close association with colleagues tended to maintain both ethical and scientific standards. The "solo" practitioner, in contrast, could become lax in these respects, since there were few checks on his work after he once secured a license. Solo practice, nevertheless, remained the rule

[106] *Medicine in the Changing Order* (New York: Report of N.Y. Acad. of Med., Commonwealth Fund, 1947), pp. 132 f.; J. E. Deitrick and R. C. Berson, eds., *Medical Schools in the United States at Mid-Century* (Evanston, Ill.: Assoc. Amer. Med. Colleges, 1960), pp. 303–8.

[107] D. G. Anderson *et al.*, "Medical Education in the United States and Canada," *Jour. of the Amer. Med. Assoc.*, vol. 150 (Sept. 13, 1952), p. 130; *Medicine in the Changing Order* (n. 106, above), p. 133. In 1959 it was estimated that there were about 230,000 licensed physicians in the U.S.A., see L. E. Burney, *Bull. Amer. College of Surgeons*, vol. 44 (January, 1959), pp. 9–11, 58–63.

in most parts of the country, except insofar as physicians associated with hospitals and medical schools derived thereby some of the values of group organization. At present, there is some promise in cooperative arrangements between hospitals, schools, and health departments for bringing the latest technical knowledge to doctors through television programs.[108]

[108] *Medicine in the Changing Order* (n. 106, above), p. 138.

CHAPTER III ⤫ PROBLEMS AND PROCEDURES IN LICENSING, 1900–1965

Of the three issues involving the quality of medical care mentioned above—quackery, obsolescence, and the multiplicity of licensing boards—it was in the latter area that most progress was made after 1910. Although, as noted, certain examining boards had made reciprocity arrangements by that year, the fact remained that men licensed in one state often faced additional tests upon moving into other jurisdictions. Such requirements were particularly difficult for middle-aged doctors who lacked opportunities for refresher training. Of course, difficulties should have been placed in the way of men actually obsolescent, but even competent older men found it awkward to take complete examinations all over again. Meantime, the increase in the number of states to forty-eight by 1920 did not help matters.

The suggestion that the problem might be solved by "a universal (national) practitioner's license" was revived by various physicians in 1902 and 1903—one of whom has been cited. In 1902, indeed, an editorial in the A.M.A. *Journal* suggested that the President appoint a national board of medical examiners for men seeking government appointments and it was hoped that those approved by such a board would also be accepted by the states. In the same year a conference called by the A.M.A. Committee on National Legislation, aware of the failure to agree on reciprocity, recommended that the House of Delegates approve a voluntary national board. Action on this was delayed by opposition from state boards but the latter remained unable to agree on systematic reciprocity. Proposals for a voluntary national board again appeared in the *Journal* in 1906 and in 1914, but without immediate result.

In retrospect, the proposal that the federal government set standards in medical licensing was still unrealistic. In terms of American tradition, national licensing would have to come from a voluntary medical society representing the whole country, or else from some body—also voluntary—set up expressly for this purpose. The possibility that the A.M.A. could issue a national license does not seem to have been seriously considered. The nearest approach to this was probably the suggestion of 1859 that the letters M.A.M.A. be used rather than the questionable M.D. But there is no evidence that the states would have conferred legal status on a designation of this sort, and the states, rather than the federal government, remained the final authorities in this area.

The founding of a special, voluntary agency, proposed as early as 1902, was thus the most promising expedient. Interest in this possibility increased after 1910, when medical education was being reorganized all along the line. In 1915 Dr. William L. Rodman announced, in a presidential address before the A.M.A., that a National Board of Medical Examiners had been set up during the preceding month. The House of Delegates referred the matter to the Council on Medical Education, which approved the board unanimously some months later. The council favored the plan for providing examinations which, it was hoped, would be accepted by all state boards. It was also favorably impressed (1) by the make-up of the National Board, which included representatives from the federal medical services, the Association of American Medical Colleges, the Federation of State Medical Boards, the American College of Surgeons, and the A.M.A.; (2) by assurance of adequate foundation funds for some years; and (3) by the standards proposed for applicants and for the examinations in view. These standards, high for 1915, involved:

> A diploma from a four-year high school in good standing.
> A satisfactory [arts] college course in the natural sciences.

Graduation from a Grade A medical school.
At least one year's internship in an acceptable hospital.

Limiting applicants to graduates of Grade A schools was particularly important, since this screened out mediocre candidates and added to the value of the board's certificates. This requirement may also have exerted further pressure on schools to secure an A rating.[109]

It is of interest that, meanwhile, the Dominion of Canada had encountered similar problems. The Canadians, like the Americans, had inherited a federal system from the old British Empire. But in their own blend of British and American procedures, they turned both to the national government (the British way) and to the provincial authorities (the American way) for a combined licensing program. To be specific, in 1912 a Dominion Medical Council was set up under government auspices, representing the schools and provincial colleges of physicians and surgeons. This council prepared examinations which, if passed, qualified candidates for licensing by provincial agencies—subject to supplementary requirements by the latter bodies.[110] It was not until three years later, as noted, that the voluntary National Board was organized across the border.

Several developments ensued in 1916 which assured the survival of the National Board in the United States. Guidance was secured from a joint conference held by the A.M.A. Council on Medical Education and the Federation of State Boards, and continued financial support came from the Carnegie Foun-

[109] N. A. Womack, "The Evolution of the National Board of Medical Examiners" (pamphlet), n.d., Chapel Hill, N.C., pp. 12–15.

[110] *Ibid.,* p. 16; *Quarter of a Century of Progress: Highlights of the First Twenty-five Years* (Philadelphia: Nat. Board of Med. Examiners, 1940), pp. 5–7; on Canada, see W. L. Bierring, "Medical Licensure after Forty Years," *Conn. State Med. Jour.,* vol. 20 (Sept., 1956), p. 726; and J. S. Thompson, "The Canadian Student—Western Style," *Jour. Med. Educ.,* vol. 33 (November, 1958), p. 793. I am also indebted to Dr. Lloyd Stevenson, formerly Dean, School of Medicine at McGill University, for information on Canadian developments.

dation for the Advancement of Teaching. No doubt state boards at first feared that a rival organization was being established, perhaps with the backing of federal agencies. Eight states, nevertheless, agreed at once to accept the National Board examinations. Three of these (Colorado, Idaho, and North Dakota) were western, two were in New England (New Hampshire, Vermont) and three were in or on the border of the South (Maryland, Kentucky, and North Carolina). What correlations may have existed between the first agreements and the economic or professional status of each of these states are not apparent, though it may be noted that only one—Maryland —possessed a large city with strong medical institutions.

The first National Board examinations were held in federal hospitals in Washington in 1916, when the sudden impact of high standards resulted in considerable attrition. Of thirty-two applicants, only sixteen were considered qualified; of the latter, ten actually appeared and only five passed. Both total numbers and ratios increased slowly over the next five years. In eleven examinations, 1916 to 1921, there were 498 applicants, of whom 427 were qualified and 325 appeared. Among the latter, 269 passed.

Meantime, at the close of World War I, the National Board sent two members abroad to study licensure in England, Scotland, and France. They were cordially received by professional leaders, including Sir William Osler, and five representatives of British and French licensing bodies in return visited the United States in 1920. As a result of these exchanges, the Conjoint Board in England, the Triple Qualification Board of Scotland, and the National Board in the United States agreed upon mutual acceptance of the basic parts of their respective examinations. This was an important step in advancing international medical relations and also provided the National Board with prestige at home.[111]

[111] Womack, "National Board of Medical Examiners" (n. 109, above), pp. 19 f.

Unfortunately, Dr. Rodman—founder of the board—had died in 1916, but was succeeded as secretary by his son, Dr. J. Stewart Rodman. The latter secured additional funds from the Carnegie Foundation in 1921, and also from several other large foundations. In the same year the board attained legal status by being incorporated in the District of Columbia, and employed a managing director.

In 1922 Dr. Rodman—after consultations with the foreign visitors—inaugurated those studies of examination methods which were to become a feature of the board's later history. Instead of depending largely on oral discussions and case demonstrations, as heretofore, the board now approved a three-part program. Part I was a written examination on preclinical fields, Part II a written test relating to third- and fourth-year clinical work, and Part III a practical examination in clinical and laboratory problems given at the bedside. It was necessary to pass Part I in order to take Part II, and no one could take Part III before passing Part II and completing a year's internship. Thus, the "national boards" began to be taken at intervals in the medical student's career; and Part III, involving bedside procedure, was made available at more than twenty centers throughout the country.

This was a period when professional educators and psychologists were giving increasing heed to new types of testing.[112] Whether Dr. Rodman was influenced by these trends is not clear: certainly, he was guided in part by his knowledge of medical experience. Later, both the national and state boards would employ new types of tests when these appeared useful.

Since the National Board provided superior examinations, the organization transcended its original object of convenience to candidates. It began to represent a measure of excellence

[112] In 1923 alone, e.g., a journal devoted to the teaching of history published thirteen articles on testing, whereas over the preceding twelve years it had presented only ten; see R. H. Shryock, ed., "Guide to the Materials in the . . . *Historical Outlook,* Vols., I–XVI, 1909–1925," *Historical Outlook,* XVI (December, 1925), 355–94.

which was emulated by some state boards. Gradually, the latter ceased to fear the program and even found it helpful, while ambitious young doctors came to view national certification as an honor. Under these circumstances, schools became concerned about the record of their students with the board, so that the latter influenced standards even in undergraduate medical education.

In the early 1930s certain of the specialty groups sought cooperation from the National Board, and the latter approved such efforts. The A.M.A. Council on Medical Education, however, did not support these proposals. Instead, in 1933, the Advisory Board for Medical Specialties was founded in order to provide an agency consisting entirely of specialists. Perhaps it was just as well that the National Board did not become directly involved in post-graduate training, since its own program was steadily expanding.

By 1940 the number of candidates taking its examinations had reached some 1,400 a year, about one-fourth of all medical school graduates. A total of over 14,000 candidates had pursued this program over the preceding twenty-five years, and more than 7,000 physicians were diplomats by that time. Between 1922 and 1940, twenty medical schools—including some of the strongest institutions and, parenthetically, the one surviving college for women—had each provided 250 or more candidates. Most indicative of progress was the fact that by 1940 all but five state agencies had come to accept the "National Boards," although nine states required supplementary examinations or other special arrangements.

At its twenty-fifth anniversary dinner, Dr. Alan Gregg of the Rockefeller Foundation congratulated the National Board on its work "in setting standards and in protecting the laity from those who would willingly let loose upon a trusting public the shoddy product of inadequate preparation for the practice of medicine." The implication here was clear that state boards were inadequate, indeed, Dr. Gregg referred to them as providing "an outmoded, isolated but stubborn system of local examiners."[113] This view would have shocked the medical reformers of 1875–1900 who had labored long to secure these same boards, and Dr. Gregg was probably aware of this. But he was responding to accelerating advances in medical science and perhaps also to the national drift away from "states' rights" in general. He was raising his sights and in doing so envisaged a future for the National Board.

In 1950, when Dr. Rodman was about to retire, Dr. John P. Hubbard became assistant secretary and then executive director. Dr. Hubbard was familiar with objective tests and statistical methods which had developed rapidly since the 1930s. In 1951–52, with the help of the Educational Testing Service at Princeton, objective tests were prepared for both internal medicine and for surgery. These proved so successful that similar examinations were adopted for the entire Part I and Part II programs. Panels of experts were assembled to complete the examination forms, after which they met again to study results and to prepare the next version. All told, by the 1950s, from seventy to eighty outstanding medical professors were so engaged at any one time, and these men developed a marked ability to measure medical competence. They returned to their schools, moreover, with a growing interest in teaching which probably improved these institutions.

Some state boards, it is true, objected to the substitution of objective tests for essay questions, and several withdrew approval of the national boards for this reason. In so doing, they shared the attitude of many arts-college professors who disliked true-false, multiple choice, and other testing devices which were coming into vogue. The National Board became convinced nevertheless, that the advantages of these forms—

[113] Womack, "National Board of Medical Examiners" (n. 109, above), pp. 24 f.; *Quarter of a Century of Progress* (n. 110, above), pp. 13–15, 31–39.

in brevity, in comprehensiveness, and in ease of measuring—more than compensated for the extra time needed in preparing them. Especially helpful was the elimination of much of the subjectivity involved in grading essays. In due time most state boards became reconciled to objective tests, and by 1964 only two or three of them still withheld approval of National Board certification.

The services rendered by the National Board were related, both as cause and effect, to the general improvement of the medical schools. This improvement continued into the 1930s, by which time research was advancing therapy and American physicians were beginning to receive Nobel prizes. As a result of scientific achievements, and despite a relatively low median income, public opinion surveys of the 1930s ascribed to physicians the highest standing among occupational groups.[114] In view of their low status as late as the 1880s, this position of doctors a half century later revealed them in a Cinderella role unique in the history of American professions.

It gradually became apparent, nevertheless, that the reforms of 1910–30 had by no means ushered in a medical millenium. The closing of many schools reduced the number of physicians in civilian practice from about 146,500 in 1910 to 145,000 in 1930. The proportion of doctors to population (now stated in total figures) dropped from 154 per 100,000 in 1910 to only 121 in 1930.[115] Such a decline was sure to elicit public concern, but before discussing that reaction something may be said of repercussions within the profession and within medical colleges in particular.

[114] Public opinion surveys were a product of new sampling techniques developed by statisticians and sociologists, chiefly after 1930. See, e.g., G. W. Hartman, "Prestige of Occupation," *Personnel Jour.*, XIII (October, 1934); and H. J. Walter, "The Relative Social Prestige of Twenty Professions," unpublished thesis, University of Wisconsin, 1935, pp. 23 ff.

[115] Dael Wolfle, Director, *America's Resources of Specialized Talent* . . . (New York: Harpers, 1954), pp. 106–8. There is some discrepancy between these figures and those given in patients-per-doctor ratios (n. 91, above), but not enough to affect generalizations.

The excess of applications to enter medical schools seemed at first a great advantage, in that admission committees could select only candidates with excellent premedical records in the sciences. Here and there, however, professors criticized this procedure as calculated to produce "mere technicians." Fears were expressed that the doctors of the future would lack cultural background—the very quality which had once set physicians off from less prestigious guilds. Thus, in 1931, a writer in the *Journal of the Association of American Medical Colleges* referred to students in terms reminiscent of the 1850s:

> Our students [he declared] are the most uninteresting of men. They are ignorant of either art or literature. They only read sporting pages and cheap magazines. They do not even know their own language, nor can they spell. They are, in fact, semi illiterate.[116]

There were also occasional statements that the profession still contained many men who were inadequately trained and/or unethical in conduct. Surgery was the chief target of such accusations, both because of fee-splitting and as a result of continued toleration of surgical work by general practitioners. The late General Paul Hawley, chief surgeon of the European area during World War II declared in 1959 that: "It is now widely estimated that today one-half of the surgical operations . . . are performed by doctors who are untrained, or inadequately trained, to undertake surgery." But twelve years earlier he had included the whole profession in the remark that: "had organized medicine devoted half as much energy to kicking out the rascals as it has to protecting them, there would be no danger of government control of medicine."[117] Such statements, also reminiscent of earlier comments, implied that even the more careful selection of future doctors had not kept out all "the rascals." But screening for moral qualities is a particularly elusive matter for both faculties and licensing authorities. One

---

[116] Quoted by Justin Miller, *The Philosophy of Professional Licensure* (Columbia, S.C.: Nat. Coun. State Boards of Engr. Examiners, 1937), p. 13.
[117] Obituary, *New York Times,* November 26, 1965, p. 35.

surmises—though it may be damning with faint praise—that the profession was ethically superior by the 1940s to what it had been a half century before.

Just as serious as the charge that objectionable men still slipped into the guild was the reverse indictment that many good persons were excluded. Liberals stated that ethnic or religious prejudices, especially against Negroes but also against Jews and Catholics, were increasing and were driving qualified students to European countries for training. The high tide in this migration, in 1936, carried about 2,000 individuals abroad —a number which must have exceeded any record established during the earlier trek to German universities. As usual, meanwhile, little was said about concomitant sex discrimination in admissions to American schools, although the proportion of women students continued to average about five per cent, and the ratio of women within the profession declined slightly between 1910 and 1940.[118] All such types of discrimination are difficult to prove or measure, but it is a common impression that ethnic and religious prejudices have declined over the last decade or two.

A more sweeping reaction to the reforms of 1910–30 was the view that these changes had been introduced too rapidly or perhaps carried too far. Even before some schools had been modernized, complaints were made that scientific progress combined with strict "legal requirements" (licensing) were not an unmixed blessing. By 1925 observers noted a growing resistance among faculties against applying further regulations until there was time for re-thinking and experimentation. A commission of the A.M.A. Council on Medical Education, cooperating with representatives of medical colleges and of state boards, agreed upon a truce of some years in order to permit

---

[118] See S. Jarcho, "Medical Education in the United States, 1950–1956," *Jour. Mt. Sinai Hosp.* (New York City), XVII (July, 1959), 356–60; Shryock, "Women in American Medicine" (n. 72, above), p. 377.

readjustments to the new dispensation. In consequence, the Association of American Medical Colleges (A.A.M.C.) was recognized as the standardizing agency. Under its oversight the schools were to be permitted leeway in reorganizing curricula.

During the next quarter-century, as a result of intra-professional pressures, emphasis in undergraduate curricula shifted from anatomy, pathology, and surgery (in the nineteenth-century tradition) to biochemistry, biophysics, physiology, internal medicine, and psychiatry. It was not only the curriculum, of course, which was changing: so also were nearly all aspects of medical education. Admissions, costs, faculties, relations to hospitals, post-graduate programs, and research were all undergoing modification at an increasing rate. So marked were the changes that in 1947 the A.A.M.C., with the Flexner Report of 1910 in mind, planned another general survey. The outcome was a study on medical schools in the United States at mid-century (1960), which presented a comprehensive account of trends as seen from within the schools.[119]

Even as medical colleges consolidated their own reforms, they came under pressure from extramural sources—from foundations, university officials, scientific societies—for further changes in curricula and administration. In view of an excessive maternal death rate, for example, efforts to improve the teaching and practice of obstetrics were initiated by the New York Academy of Medicine with the aid of the Commonwealth Fund.[120] Alan Gregg, acting for the Rockefeller Foundation, promoted the teaching of psychiatry. Meantime, with the encouragement of presidents or trustees, medical schools—except

[119] Rappleye, "Major Changes in Medical Education" (n. 90, above), pp. 685–88. Deitrick and Berson, *Medical Schools at Mid-Century* (n. 106, above), was published by the A.A.M.C.

[120] Esther L. Brown, *Physicians and Medical Care* (New York: Russell Sage Foundation, 1937), pp. 38–44; J. F. Rogers, "The Last Fifty Years," *N.Y. State Jour. of Med.*, vol. 57 (February, 1957), pp. 495–97.

for the few independent colleges—gave up some autonomy and moved toward integration with their respective universities. They also sought a closer relationship with society at large, as in presenting social and environmental medicine and in a cautious insertion of behavioral science into the curriculum. In the latter case also, the initiative sometimes came from without rather than from within the medical institutions.

The introduction of social-science outlooks was, at first, more important than the advent of formal courses. At Johns Hopkins, Henry Sigerist presented medical history from a social perspective in the early 1930s, and at about the same time sociologists and economists became interested in the current relations of medicine and society. Some were concerned with the economics of medical care, some with social medicine (social factors in disease), and still others with the sociology of medical professions and institutions. It was not easy to integrate the thinking of behavioral scientists and of biologically trained physicians, but within the medical setting specialists in preventive medicine, in public hygiene, and in psychiatry were inclined to cooperate.[121]

Some medical men listened, also, to what sociologists had to say about interpersonal relationships among patients, doctors, and nurses, or about the implications of the hospital environment for both patients and staff. Of some interest were studies of the effects of medical education on the attitudes of students.[122] After 1950 the Russell Sage Foundation, of which

[121] See Roemer, *Sigerist on Sociology of Medicine* (n. 15, above); e.g., the article therein "The Special Position of the Sick" (Leipzig, 1929), which lacks the current data employed by sociologists, but provides depth in time lacking in most sociologic studies. On the introduction of professional sociology, see L. S. Cottrell, Jr. and Eleanor B. Sheldon, "Problems of Collaboration between Social Scientists and the Practicing Professions," *Annals* (n. 122, below), pp. 127–37.

[122] See, e.g., E. L. Brown, *Newer Dimensions of Patient Care* (New York: Russell Sage Foundation, Pt. I, 1961; Pt. II, 1962); S. W. Bloom, "The Process of Becoming a Physician," *Annals of the Amer. Acad. of Polit. and Soc. Sci.,* vol. 346 (March, 1963), pp. 82–86.

Dr. Donald Young was director, encouraged the application of behavioral science to the training of the chief professions, and sociologists and anthropologists appeared in consequence in certain medical and public health institutions across the country.[123]

At about this time interest in methods of teaching was encouraged by the Association of Medical Colleges. Such interest also may have reflected a general enthusiasm for progressive education (1915 to 1940). One aspect of this was a growing awareness of the value of self-training for the student—a view fore-shadowed at Hopkins as early as 1893. Residencies seemed made to order for self-education, but the first step toward these posts—internship, which fell between undergraduate and post-graduate programs—became a subject of some concern.

The problem was that about two-thirds of internships were located in non-university hospitals—which were usually non-teaching hospitals. These institutions valued interns largely for their immediate aid and were unwilling or unable to provide the further clinical training for which this service had been planned. (The situation seemed analogous to the exploitation of student nurses in some hospitals.) In consequence, medical colleges were urged to make teaching arrangements in as many hospitals as possible, or at least to retain oversight of the "fifth year" in the educational sequence.[124] Some superior hospitals not connected with schools, it should be added, gave attention to clinical teaching on their own initiative.

By the 1950s readjustments in undergraduate programs not only involved shifts in curricula and teaching methods but also, in certain schools, basic reorganizations. Thus, at Western

[123] An overview of this whole field and of the extensive, recent literature is S. H. King's *Perceptions of Illness and Medical Practice* (New York: Russell Sage Foundation, 1962).

[124] Esther E. Lape, ed., *American Medicine: Expert Testimony out of Court* (New York: Amer. Foundation, 1937), pp. 390–92; *Medicine in the Changing Order* (n. 106, above), p. 130.

Reserve University (Cleveland) students had been placed in hospital services as early as the first two years during the 1930s, and in the 1950s the curriculum was planned in relation to organic systems rather than in terms of traditional subjects. Late in the same decade concern about the time factor and also about isolation from the humanities led The Johns Hopkins medical school to introduce an experimental system. Under this arrangement selected students could be admitted after two years in college but carried on further work in the arts under the control of the medical faculty. One effect was to shorten the total course of arts and medical training by a year or two—usually to seven years.

In 1961 even more radical departures were made at Northwestern and at Boston University, which returned to the pattern of admission directly from high schools, and so reduced the time sequence still further. At Boston, the entire class could be admitted on this basis. Like Hopkins, these schools provided some arts training, but they placed less emphasis on student research and electives than did the Baltimore institution. Equally radical experimentation is to be expected in the fourteen new medical schools now (in 1965) in process of development.[125]

The planning of additional schools was a response to renewed imbalance between the need for and supply of physicians. Here was another respect in which the reforms of 1910–20 were carried too far, since the decline in the number of medical colleges and their graduates continued into the 1930s despite population expansion. During that decade some physicians still held that there were too many doctors, but others had their doubts. As a member of a California group summed it up about 1935: "Since 1904 our medical graduates have been

---

[125] P. V. Lee, *Medical Schools and the Changing Times . . .,* (Evanston, Ill.: Assoc. Amer. Med. Colleges, 1962), pp. 5–9; *The AMA News,* Nov. 15, 1965, pp. 1, 11.

reduced fifty percent through a period when there has been great increase in our population. This is basically wrong."[126] Professional leaders became openly worried by the situation in the 1940s, when school enrollments declined because of World War II and when it seemed improbable that additional faculties could be recruited without lowering standards.

The whole problem was complicated by a maldistribution of doctors, who were becoming increasingly scarce in general practice and in rural areas.[127] It also appeared that there never had been enough psychiatrists. That a general shortage was developing, moreover—in terms of services desired—could not be doubted. One way of illustrating this is to note that the number of approved residencies in hospitals increased 600 per cent between 1940 and 1960, while the output of medical graduates rose only 35 per cent. In other words, the schools had done much to increase demand for specialized hospital care, but were unable to turn out enough men to provide this care. More will be said on this theme later. It may be added that after 1950 a shortage of registered nurses became even more serious than that of physicians.[128]

The very fact that there were not enough medical schools may have increased the prestige of existing institutions. The reputation of medical faculties, moreover, made them a dynamic factor in raising the status of the whole profession. Professors were in demand not only as consultants but also for service on boards, surveys, commissions, and the like. An increasing proportion of them gave up, or never entered, private practice. Such men became more distinct from practitioners than medical teachers had been a half century before—in which respect they

---

[126] Lape, *American Medicine* (n. 124, above), pp. 8–14.

[127] See F. D. Mott and M. I. Roemer, *Rural Health and Medical Care* (New York: McGraw-Hill, 1948), chap. 8.

[128] *Medicine in the Changing Order* (n. 106, above), pp. 124–26; 189–96; A. C. Eurich, "The Citizen's Health: Whose Responsibility?", *Saturday Review,* Oct. 28, 1961, pp. 14–16.

followed the path of German professors during that earlier period. One could, in some cases, note this trend in subtle distinctions made between full-time and part-time staff. The former might now identify themselves more with universities or research institutes than with medical societies.

It is not strange, under these circumstances, that schools displayed a growing independence of the societies. In the early 1900s part-time professors had been leaders within the A.M.A. in persuading that body to reform medical colleges, but between 1920 and 1940 the views of full-time academic doctors often diverged from those of most practitioners. (The A.M.A., for example, followed constituent societies after 1920 in opposing compulsory health insurance, but many professors maintained a liberal stand on this issue.[129]) In view of the total situation, some critics decided that standards as well as policies should again be entrusted to the schools rather than to conservative societies. Was there not need once more for freedom in educational experiments? As a committee of the New York Academy of Medicine put it in 1947:

> Licensure by state boards was highly desirable when the standards observed in most schools were very low. At the present time, however, the system . . . tends to keep the medical curriculum rigid. . . . Now that relatively high standards are maintained in most schools, it is desirable to return the licensing power to them in order that they may be free to experiment with the curriculum.[130]

The Academy's committee added, however, that if licensing by schools was not revived, there would be "obvious advantages in countrywide acceptance of some universal standard for licensure." It was in that direction, with the continued growth of the National Board of Medical Examiners, that licensure

---

[129] See *Jour. of the Amer. Med. Assoc.,* vol. 109 (Oct. 16, 1937), pp. 1280 ff. New York *Herald Tribune,* Nov. 6, 1937; Esther Lape, "Medical Education as discussed in 'American Medicine,' " *Jour. Assoc. Amer. Med. Colleges,* XII (November, 1937), pp. 359 ff.

[130] *Medicine in the Changing Order* (n. 106, above), p. 131; see also Lape, *American Medicine* (n. 124, above), pp. 454–56.

was actually moving. As noted, by 1940 the candidates taking its examinations had reached some 1,400 a year—about one-fourth of the medical school graduates—and by 1964 the numbers taking national boards increased ten-fold to about 14,000 a year. As before, scientists and clinicians spent many hours in creating examinations which now involved a total of five days (thirty hours) of testing.

During such planning, experiments were made with more sophisticated techniques. Particularly difficult was the preparation of checks on clinical ability. It proved impossible, for example, to provide uniform tests in surgery, so that there was an inclination to leave rating to the chiefs of services in which candidates had been trained. (In effect, a vestige of licensing by the schools.) On the other hand, the problem of presenting a uniform test in internal medicine—diagnosis and therapy—was solved in an ingenious manner. Since it would have been invalid to test candidates throughout the country by confronting them with different patients, the identical case was presented by use of a moving picture including sound. Thus each variable except the student himself was eliminated.[131]

As the specialties grew in prestige more and more graduates viewed the internship as a step toward specialization. By the 1960s about 85 per cent of graduates aspired to specialization and there was in consequence a further erosion of the ranks of "family doctors." One attempt to check the latter tendency was made in setting up an academy of general practice. Meantime, some observers suggested that the schools should take over the certifying of specialists, on the ground that the latter's training was a form of post-graduate education. However, the universities showed no inclination to undertake this responsibility, so that it remained with the specialty boards.[132]

[131] *Examinations and Their Role in Evaluation and Qualification for Practice* (Philadelphia: Nat. Board of Med. Examiners, 1964), pp. ii, 38, 49, 53, 65, 102 ff. On the new clinical tests in particular, see therein J. P. Hubbard, "Programmed Testing," pp. 102–14, and the articles following.

[132] *Ibid.,* p. 49.

The universities, moreover, made no attempt to recover licensing authority in general. The matter was a delicate one, since state boards continued to be supported by medical societies, and the latter—perhaps remembering the era before 1910—were not inclined to return the function to college faculties. Dr. Morris Fishbein, as editor of the A.M.A. *Journal,* took this position openly. The A.M.A. represented state societies, and the latter were usually led by prominent physicians who, although associated with hospitals, were not full-time professors. It was this type of practitioner which, always influential, came after 1920 into almost full control of the A.M.A. Seen in short perspective, this trend has been viewed as a shift from a first generation of professional liberalism to a second generation of conservatism.[133] Actually, however, conservatives have dominated organized medicine from the founding of the A.M.A. in 1847 down to the 1960s, except for the short interval of "medical reform" in 1900–20.

During the decade following World War II, medical schools attracted a declining proportion of outstanding college graduates. It seems unlikely that this shift reflected any decline in the prestige of medicine, and the average, real income of practitioners was rising. Nevertheless competition with other professions, notably with physical scientists, lessened the relative appeal of medical careers. Not only were achievements in physics and engineering dramatic but training in these areas was neither so lengthy nor so costly as in medicine. During 1962–63, for example, about 68 per cent of all students in graduate schools (including those in the humanities) received non-refundable grants averaging $2,450. In the same year

[133] Talcott Parsons views the liberal element as the "first generation" of AMA leadership which lost control to conservatives after 1930; "Social Change and Medical Perspective," *Annals Amer. Acad. of Polit. and Soc. Science,* vol. 346 (March, 1963), pp. 31–33.

only 17 per cent of medical students were so aided, by grants averaging but $585.[134]

It seems strange, in retrospect, that greater efforts were not made to reduce the expenses faced by medical students. Foundations made gifts to medical schools as such but did little to provide fellowships or loan funds for undergraduates. Much the same thing may be said of university trustees, although charges made by state colleges were lower than those required by private institutions. One can only speculate about the reasons for seeming discrimination against medical neophytes. Perhaps the public image of graduate students in the arts was that of impecunious youth always needing help—of itinerant scholars, extending some modern equivalent of begging bowls. Medical beginners, conversely, were pictured as headed toward wealth even if temporarily poor. It seemed likely, in consequence, that future physicians would be drawn largely from the prosperous classes. Here, again, the reforms of 1910–20 may have gone too far: it had been easier for poor boys to secure professional training prior to that era.

In any case, financing education posed a greater problem for medical men than for graduate students in arts and sciences. Some efforts were made to counteract these disadvantages. Thus, a little income was at last provided for interns as well as for residents, and—as noted—certain schools reduced the total length of undergraduate education. Meantime, modest loan funds were made available to medical students by the A.M.A. and by other medical societies. These expedients were doubtless helpful, but the fact that able men continued to enter medical schools could be ascribed chiefly to increases in real income within the population and also the excess of good applicants long available. On the negative side, moreover, tests

---

[134] *Datagrams* (Evanston, Ill.: Assoc. Amer. Med. Colleges, January, 1965), vol. 6, no. 7.

for keeping out low-grade applicants were well developed by this time.

Hence the chief professional threat did not relate to the quality of students but rather to the converging of two trends already mentioned. The first was the shortage of graduates needed in hospitals and ultimately in practice, and the second was a demand for more medical care per capita. In consequence, something of a professional vacuum appeared about 1935 and expanded after 1950. Into this void moved physicians from abroad.

Strictly speaking, the first such group to arrive had been the German refugees of 1848. Next, during the 1920s, Americans who had secured foreign degrees returned to take state boards —and many of them failed. By the 1930s a second wave of political refugees arrived from Germany and certain of these men thought they were discriminated against in state examinations. Soon thereafter some European and Canadian doctors, impressed by the financial prospects or by the growing prestige of American medicine, sought residencies or other hospital posts in this country. They were analogous to Americans who had taken advanced training in Germany until 1914, except that some planned to remain here rather than to return to their homeland.

It was after World War II, also, that non-European doctors were first attracted to the United States in large numbers. The quality of their training was uncertain. Upon arrival, these men found that state boards required training in an American hospital and they therefore sought internships in order to qualify for examinations. Many hospitals, short of native interns, accepted the foreign applicants even though there was no way of evaluating educational backgrounds. In New York City, most exposed to this professional invasion, more than one-third of 2,000 staff doctors employed in municipal hospitals in 1960 were immigrants of questionable training.

Some of these men, naturally enough, had language difficulties in addition to other limitations. The resulting situation suddenly threatened licensing standards developed during preceding decades. In order to study the problem a joint committee representing the Federation of State Boards, the Association of American Medical Colleges, the American Hospital Association, and the A.M.A. Council on Medical Education and Hospitals was appointed in 1954 to devise "an effective mechanism for measuring educational attainment in the absence of intimate . . . knowledge of the educational background of foreign physicians." In response to the joint committee's findings the four bodies set up in 1957 the Educational Council for Foreign Medical Graduates (E.C.F.M.G.). This agency, operating under trustees representing the sponsors, was aided financially by the Kellogg and the Rockefeller foundations and appointed a full-time staff in Evanston, Illinois.

The purposes of the new council were to extend information about American requirements, and also to enable qualified men to secure E.C.F.M.G. certification before applying for appointments or examinations in the United States. In order to implement certification, the National Board of Medical Examiners (N.B.M.E.) was asked to aid in providing a screening examination. The National Board agreed, and the E.C.F.M.G. gave its first examinations in 1958. During the next few months Dr. Hubbard, director of the board, visited medical centers throughout the world and was able to arrange that these examinations be given abroad as well as in this country. The procedure was made possible through the cooperation of American embassies.

The scale of the program in which the N.B.M.E. was thus involved is indicated by the fact that in one of two examinations given in 1963, over 10,750 individuals took the E.C.F.M.G. examinations in English as well as in technical subjects—a year during which the total candidates from approved American schools numbered about 14,400. In 1962 the number of foreign candidates taking the examinations abroad began to exceed those in this country, and the proportion of the former group reached about 71 per cent by 1963. There were, at first, a large number of failures, and this compelled the withdrawal from certain hospitals of many physicians trained abroad. The situation improved somewhat as the E.C.F.M.G. program became well established, and over the years, between 1958 and 1963, about three-fifths of foreign applicants were eventually certified.[135]

The foreign supply, however, was not adequate to make up for the shortage of native physicians. In 1958, all told, the country had about 230,000 licensed practitioners. This number provided (for a total population of about 170 million) a ratio of roughly one doctor for 740 persons—as compared to 1:600 in 1900, and 1:763 in 1938. The proportion of doctors was thus slightly higher in 1958 than it had been twenty years earlier, but several facts should be recalled in this connection. Population expansion had slowed down during the 1930s, encouraging the idea that the decline in medical graduates had not been excessive, but by the 1950s an increase in the birth rate threatened to upset the doctor-patient balance seriously.

Whether or not the ratio of about 1:740 was considered adequate in 1958, the population growth of the early 1960s so accelerated that the maintenance of this proportion became problematical. It was estimated that to maintain then current ratios would require an increase in the number of new doctors and dentists each year from 12,500 in 1962 to 19,000 in 1970. Yet it would cost at least $30 million and from five to ten

---

[135] Womack, "Evolution of National Board of Medical Examiners" (n. 109, above), pp. 28–30; Eurich, "The Citizen's Health" (n. 128, above), p. 15; *Jour. of Med. Educ.*, vol. 33 (February, 1958), p. xviii; "Medical Licensure Statistics for 1963," (annual report of AMA council on medical education), *Jour. of the Amer. Med. Assoc.*, vol. 188 (June 8, 1964), pp. 885–900.

years in time to found one additional school—which could then provide only 100 more doctors a year.[136]

The fact was that the ratio of 1:740, even if adequate in 1958, was no longer satisfactory for 1962 and was likely to be less so by 1970. In the first place, therapy became more promising and public desire for medical services mounted in consequence. In 1930 the average person had made about 2.5 visits to a doctor annually; by 1959 this figure had risen to 5.3.[137] The trend was encouraged not only by prospects of effective treatment but also by ability to pay for more service through health insurance. The demand for national medical care (compulsory health insurance) had been revived in the 1930s but was blocked for more than three decades by the return of prosperity and by the opposition of the A.M.A. In consequence, voluntary insurance expanded rapidly.

During the 1950s and 1960s, moreover, federal programs in aid of medical education and hospitals gained considerable headway. This trend reflected scientific progress as well as a continued concern for social security. Early in the century, nearly all lives saved through medical service were still those of children; by the 1940s, adults were also becoming beneficiaries. In the early 1960s average life expectancy at birth edged up to about 70 years and there was a consequent increase in the ratio of older people to total population. Many of the elderly were too poor to afford voluntary health insurance, and the drive for national insurance was most easily focused on this old-age group. President Kennedy supported such a program in 1962 but it died in Congress. Under President Johnson's leadership in 1965, however, the "Medicare" bill—assuring

---

[136] C. Taeuber and Irene B. Taeuber, *The Changing Population of the United States* (New York: John Wiley, 1958), pp. 315–18; Howard Rusk, "Doctor Shortage Grows," *New York Times,* Oct. 14, 1962; H. Nelson, "New Medical Programs . . .," *Philadelphia Inquirer,* Dec. 5, 1965, section F.

[137] Eurich, "The Citizen's Health" (n. 128, above), p. 14.

"free" hospital care and also low-cost, voluntary insurance against doctors' bills—was adopted by the federal government.

Thus, about fifty years after the reforms of the Flexner era, national medical care was approved for part of the civilian population. The time lag here was about the same as the interval which had elapsed in the United Kingdom between the medical reform bill of 1858 and the first stage of compulsory health insurance adopted in 1911.

In the United States, as in other lands, the passage of such legislation was part of an expanding social security program, and in this country, as earlier in Europe, the provision of free medical care was apt to increase demand for services. In this respect, the timing of Medicare seemed unfortunate: in addition to the general shortage of medical personnel, some doctors and nurses were being diverted into military assignments. In view of European precedents, moreover, the advent of governmental programs for part of the population was likely to presage state medicine on a still larger scale. If so, the personnel problem might become alarming.

Confronted by these uncertainties journalists called public attention to all aspects of medical care. They rediscovered issues which had been discussed by doctors and social scientists for decades, and popular articles proliferated in newspapers and in such magazines as *Life, Look, The Atlantic, The New Yorker,* and *Greater Philadelphia.* Most of these analyzed a particular problem such as hospital services, but there were also reviews of trends all along the medical front. Much of this literature held the A.M.A. responsible for current difficulties, though there were also claims that the Democratic administration had "failed tragically" to prepare for the new federal system. Somewhat reassuring, in contrast, was an estimate by the American Hospital Association, that Medicare would result in demands for a seven per cent increase in patient beds—a situation which would embarrass only those institutions which ran essentially full at all times.

When Medicare went into operation in July, 1966, there was no actual rush into hospitals and newspaper headlines were reassuring. After all, a significant proportion of elderly persons had been receiving medical services before this act was passed. Some observers warned, however, that mid-summer was a relatively healthy period and that demands might rise toward year's end. In any event no final conclusions about the impact of the new law could be formed during the first six months of its operation. As implied, many problems were involved, among which none was more vital than the probable shortage of physicians and of ancillary personnel.

So alarming was this prospect that proposals were made to revert to the training of "junior" practitioners—not to care for the masses (as in earlier days) but rather to provide services not requiring the aid of fully-trained doctors. Arrangements for this purpose had long existed in certain undeveloped countries such as Fiji, where they had evolved as a first stage in introducing Western medicine in the absence of physicians. But such a program, analogous to that for public health nurses in isolated regions, was no longer geared into the professional situation in the United States. It had been assumed that the increasing number of assistants (technicians, and physical therapists), as well as the assignment of more technical duties to nurses, had taken up most of the slack in medical practice. Yet with the threat of an increased demand for doctors and nurses, the call for partially-trained men was not surprising.

The case for training "junior-grade" doctors became stronger when related to the lack of general practitioners—a shortage not revealed in figures for the total number of physicians. Moreover, as was often pointed out, the time of the few "G.P.s" was largely taken up with minor ills. Such cases could be handled by partially-trained men—or perhaps by nurses with advanced training—who would presumably know when to refer an estimated 10 per cent of patients to colleagues holding an M.D.

Partial education could involve at least two years' work in the usual medical college or perhaps in a hospital-school planned for this purpose. The latter would cost less to set up than would a standard medical institution. It could revive the M.B. degree for graduates who would practice under some supervision from a preceptor or within a group unit. Arrangements might be made, meantime, for granting promising junior-grade men or women an M.D., after experience or further education was acquired—a return to the earliest provisions for a degree in this country.

These proposals merited consideration, since the lack of general practitioners was a serious matter. On the other hand, difficulties could be envisaged. Outside of group practice or of hospital units, could "assistant doctors" be effectively supervised? Would well-educated patients consult them as long as M.D.s were available? If not, their practice might be largely among the poor at relatively low fees. And this situation would involve a return to low-grade service for low-income families, unless comprehensive health insurance were provided. True, a program for "assistants" might enable some students to enter medicine who otherwise could not afford the costs. But would not better men of this type push on rapidly to full-M.D. status, thus leaving a residue of mediocrity on the junior level?

It semed wise, therefore, to experiment with such a program before deciding to adopt it on a large scale. (Duke University trained a few "physicians' assistants" in 1965–66, through a two-year, post-high school sequence.) Meantime, various other plans were undertaken for expanding medical personnel: the improvement of high schools, an extended recruitment of technicians, the reduction of arts-college premedical requirements, financial assistance to medical students and the provision of new four-year medical schools. Also indicated were efforts to use hospital and nursing-home facilities more effectively. In consequence of these activities, the ratio of physicians to population rose from about 1:740 in 1958 to 1:700 in 1965. As noted, however, the proportion of generalists within the profession continued to decline. The recruitment of women as physicians, moreover, continued to be neglected.[138]

The relationship of surviving medical sects to personnel problems was none too clear. One may surmise that osteopaths, as their schools improved, provided, in effect, second-grade general practitioners. Although "regulars" long repudiated such men in principle, the need for them was again recognized by some doctors in the 1960s. Osteopaths, however, were independent "doctors" subject to no routine supervision, and by the 1950s showed signs of following homeopaths back into orthodox medicine. If the former are absorbed, even as the latter, they also are likely to turn to specialization as soon as their outlook merges with that of the regular profession.

It is interesting to speculate, finally, on the role which midwives might play in meeting future needs for practitioners. Here was a guild whose historic experience had just reversed that of doctors. As specialists, they had been partially replaced by general practitioners after 1800, and their ranks were further depleted during the present century as a result of economic trends and of sharp criticisms aimed at them by obstetricians. Meantime, midwives received improved training in some Euro-

---

[138] Nelson, "New Medical Programs" (n. 136, above). See also D. Stetten in "Medicine in the Year 2000" (n. 105, above), p. 105, *re* women doctors; and L. Hellman, "Let's Use Midwives—to Save Babies," *Sat. Eve. Post,* Nov. 21, 1964, pp. 8, 10. On programs in undeveloped countries, see E. F. Rosinski and F. J. Spencer, *The Assistant Medical Officer* . . . (Chapel Hill: Univ. of N.C. Press, 1965), *passim.* On recruitment, note also "Manpower for Research . . ., 1965–1970," Resources for Medical Research, Report no. 3, U.S. Pub. Health Serv., Bethesda, Md. (January, 1963), pp. 35 f.; J. Spivak; *re* nurses, in *Wall Street Jour.* (Jan. 17, 26, 1967); and J. Z. Bowers, "Women in Medicine . . .," *New Eng. Jour. of Med.,* vol. 275 (Aug. 18, 1966), pp. 362–65, *re* lack of women as physicians.

pean countries where they provided supervised service in terms of specialization rather than of general practice. But only a small proportion of American doctors saw in midwifery a means for expanding medical personnel.

One may conclude the discussion of personnel problems with the comment that—in the long run—an excess of physicians encouraged training and licensing bodies to tighten requirements, and vice versa. But this supply-and-demand process usually lagged far behind need. From 1850 to 1900, it did not shut off the excess supply of doctors, and from 1930 to 1950, it did not step up production when this was indicated. In the 1950s and early 1960s, however, when appeals for more doctors became urgent, the supply-demand machinery apparently did increase recruitment by lowering standards. Recall the enlistment of questionable foreign doctors and suggestions about partially-trained practitioners.

At this point, however, cumulative improvement in examining and licensing methods (1915–65) provided means for checking any automatic threat to quality of services. Here was a planned though voluntary arrangement capable of fairly prompt action, as was apparent in dealing with foreign candidates. Outcomes could be altered, of course, if the state or public opinion blocked the best judgment of faculties and of boards.

CHAPTER IV ❧ CONCLUSIONS

The complexity of this subject may have made the preceding account diffuse at times. Or an interest in tangential issues may have disrupted continuity. To compensate if possible for such lapses, final comments are added here. Some offer interpretations which, if not new, at least differ in emphasis from commonly held views. Others are posed as questions still difficult to answer. It is hoped that these conclusions, although providing no summary of content, may bring certain themes into focus.

Let us begin with matters which, minor in themselves, are of passing interest, if not passing strange. There are, for example, certain traditions about the medical profession which seem exaggerated, though not entirely untrue—a sort of folklore which persists among both laymen and physicians. An illustration is the tradition that the old-time family doctor was a helpful and reliable man. He has become, in current terms, something of a father figure. Although the degree of truth in this view never can be measured, probabilities might be estimated if answers could be found for such questions as: (1) Does the tradition apply equally well to the doctor of 1750, of 1850, and of 1900? (2) What is meant by "helpful"? and (3) Have we sometimes idealized early medical men, in contrast to the limitations—real or fancied—of their present successors?

Space does not permit adequate answers here but, stated briefly, I have found little evidence to support the tradition mentioned. Except in the case of a few able and devoted doctors, most easily observed in large towns, we seem to be dealing here more with nostalgia than with reality. Many general practitioners, prior to 1900, had received a mediocre education at best. Yet patients were either unaware of this fact or considered it irrelevant. Indeed, the view that "practical" men need not be carefully trained and licensed was long an obstacle to the development of a learned profession in this country.[139]

Another exaggerated tradition was maintained by doctors themselves; namely, that in old times the guild was highly honored but fell into disrepute in later days. Such opinions were often voiced during the era 1840–70, and were occasionally heard as late as the present century.[140]   The element of truth here was the fact that some patients abandoned "regulars" in favor of "sectarians," and also that open criticism of the former became more common by mid-century. But it does not follow that the general reputation of practitioners was any lower in 1850 than it had been in 1800. Distrust of medical men had always been present and may simply have become more vocal because of changing circumstances. A variation on the theme was the view that patients had confidence in their own doctors but disdained the profession as a whole.[141]

The reference to prestige leads into a more significant question. Granting that the medical profession was reformed after 1900, does it necessarily follow that it had deteriorated during the preceding era? True, there is some evidence to this effect. Certain standards in the earliest schools were lowered, many

[139] See note 8, above, so far as scholars are concerned. Few manuscripts of rank-and-file practitioners survive, but there are published recollections by later doctors which express the sincere but exaggerated praise noted above. See, e.g., Carl E. Black, "Medical Practitioners in Illinois before Hard Roads," in *Essays in Honor of David J. Davis, M.D., Ph.D.* (Urbana: Univ. of Illinois Press, 1965), pp. 27–51.

[140] N. 54, above.

[141] See, e.g., F. G. Crookshank, "The Doctors and the Public," *Forum,* vol. 82 (1929), p. 22; R. S. Ferguson, "Doctor-Patient Relationships and 'Functional Illness,'" *Practitioner,* vol. 176 (1956), pp. 656–62; O. von Mering and L. W. Earley, "Major Changes in the Western Environment," *Archives of General Psychiatry,* vol. 13 (September, 1965), pp. 195–201. *Re* contrasts between public and private image of doctors, cf. Shryock, "Public Relations" (n. 43, above), pp. 321–24, and J. Bird, "Your Doctor and the A.M.A.," *Sat. Eve. Post,* Jan. 1, 1966, p. 14. Opinion of doctors was also reflected in fiction: they were main characters in some 140 novels (1870–1955), E. R. Wilbanks, "The Physician in the American Novel . . .," *Bull. of Bibliography,* vol. 22 (Sept.–Dec., 1958), pp. 164–68.

new schools were inferior, and state licensing controls (adopted 1790–1820) were later abandoned (1820–50). Some physicians, as noted, lamented the declining status of the guild. Unfortunate as all this was in itself, the story nevertheless may be interpreted in just the opposite manner. Most regular practitioners in towns, by 1850, had probably received some formal training. Even in rural Tennessee in the sample cited above,[142] this was true of nearly 50 per cent. By contrast, Toner's estimate for Virginia in the eighteenth century was only about 11 per cent.[143] And although any sort of chartered school could license graduates by 1850, the fact remains that fifty years before that date the great majority of "doctors" had received no formal training whatever.

What apparently happened was that the better physicians— perhaps comparing American schools unfavorably with European—hoped that the states would assure such standards as the British were coming to expect of apothecaries (general practitioners). But in raising their sights, these leaders not only looked down on the contemporary scene but forgot that the preceding era had put up with even lower requirements. A few observers realized this. Dr. Thomas Minor of Yale, for example, declared in 1839 that practitioners had "greatly improved" since 1800. And nearly forty years later, Dr. E. H. Clarke of Harvard stated that American doctors had become "as well equipped for practical work" as were English apothecaries.[144] In other words, although the former were not the equals of university-trained physicians abroad, they were by implication better prepared than had been their predecessors. If the medical men of 1850 or 1875 were not the father figures of tradition, neither were they as inferior as reformers assumed.

[142] N. 47, above.

[143] J. M. Toner, *Contributions to the Annals of Medical Progress in the United States, before and during the War for Independence* (Washington: 1874), p. 106.

[144] N. 82, above, for Minor's opinion; see also Clarke, "Practical Medicine," in *A Century of American Medicine* (Philadelphia: 1876), p. 19.

One may even conclude that a slow upgrading of most practitioners began (as in Britain) as early as about 1820, rather than only with the end of the century, as is often assumed.

There remains, nevertheless, the obvious query: Why was improvement so long delayed? There are plausible answers for the colonial period. Towns of some size had to appear before medical faculties could be established, and lacking these, formal education could only be secured abroad. Such training was too expensive for all but a select few. Even as late as 1810, after several native schools had been founded, educational facilities were anything but adequate. And as long as there were few schools, it was difficult to enforce or even to define licensing standards. Medical societies did secure some authority along these lines after 1780, but most of these state groups were not well-established or influential bodies.

At this point the claim that American society lacked values provided by old, prestigious bodies probably has some validity. Antiquated as were the privileges of medical corporations in Europe in the 1790s—and in Britain as late as 1850—these institutions did exert some control over licensing standards. And on the Continent, between 1800 and 1850, guild corporations were replaced by the state, which finally required university training and government examinations for all candidates in medicine. But in the American Union, the federal system and devotion to states' rights prevented the central government from taking over as in Europe.

This situation left licensing in the hands of the states, which in turn delegated it to medical societies in the British manner. But the societies, less influential than the corporations of the mother country, soon lost control to the medical schools—just when those institutions seemed to be deteriorating. Whether intervention by the national government would have slowly improved matters—as it did in the United Kingdom after 1858 —is difficult to say. If so "states' rights" was the villain of the piece, and it is ironic that Americans had not invented this tradition but simply inherited it from the British Empire.

However pertinent this interpretation may be, other influences were certainly involved. Why did state governments, possessing unquestioned authority, grant *de facto* licensing powers to inferior colleges? The lack of federal laws did not force this policy on the states. The latter were responding, rather, to circumstances inherent in American culture as a whole. One need refer, in passing, only to such matters as (1) the lack of traditional restraints; (2) indifference to science which promised no immediate utility; (3) the self-assurance of democratic folk, who assumed that they—quite as well as learned bodies—could judge professional standards; (4) the apparent analogy between religious freedom and freedom for medical sects; and (5) weaknesses in American education, notably the failure to establish real universities which could have set goals for medical schools.

This failure had derived partly from the limitations of the English tradition, partly from the difficulty of adjusting that tradition to colonial circumstances, and partly from the attitudes of Americans just noted. In the long run, American medicine had to wait upon the scientific progress of 1850–1900—particularly in France and in Germany—to transmit a stimulus which overcame the retarding factors mentioned. (The most practical of peoples could appreciate "the wonders of modern medicine.") Or, more exactly, it was the impact of this new science upon a country waxing populous and wealthy which provided the conditions essential to long-delayed medical reform.

There is no question that such reform accelerated after 1910. Yet this soon led, in turn, to a claim that the whole process had been carried too far.[145] In consequence, various adjustments

[145] For a picture of the resulting disquietude within the hitherto buoyant profession of the 1930s and 1940s, see Marion K. Sanders, *The Crisis in American Medicine* (New York: Harper, 1961), *passim* (originally in *Harpers* [magazine], October, 1960).

involved a partial return to usages abandoned only two or three generations before. Certain of these reversions have been noted, for example: (1) experiments with apprenticeships (despite clinical training now given in hospitals) ; (2) pleas to revive the preparation of supplementary, second-grade practitioners (despite the aid doctors received by this time from ancillary personnel) ;[146] (3) plans for reducing the length of premedical training (despite the complex nature of the curriculum) ; and (4) efforts to found additional schools. Most of these measures were intended to turn out more practitioners, which was just the reverse of professional objectives a half century before.

It was not necessarily true, however, that there was a shortage in all types of doctors by 1950. The continued activity of general practitioners in surgery, for example, seemed to prevent any lack of men working in this field. If such practice was dangerous, however, there arose a problem long basic in licensing. To put it bluntly: Was the service of partially-trained personnel better than no service at all? Involved in this dilemma at one time or another were second-grade doctors and nurses, as well as men practicing surgery who had had no special training therein.[147] No answer could be given to so broad a question, since much depended on the circumstances and safeguards in any given situation. Yet the question was unavoidable at times, and had to be met as relevant problems arose.

Reference to specialization raises another point of historical interest. Today, in speaking of specialization, we refer to an arrangement within one profession. But this profession itself originated in the merging of older guilds. These groups, although not specialists in the modern sense, represented distinct

---

[146] Note, e.g., statements of Dr. J. Gershon-Cohen, Einstein Med. Center, Philadelphia, that reform went too far in 1918 in abolishing schools [and students], and that a personnel similar to Russian *feldshers* will be needed when "Medicare" begins to function; *Phila. Evening Bulletin,* August 10, 1965, and April 10, 1966.

[147] This problem in surgery is discussed above, see n. 101.

traditions; notably those of physicians, of surgeons, and of apothecaries. Vestiges of this earlier situation appear in the survival of still other practitioners—dentists, pharmacists, midwives—who were true specialists and partly for that reason were not incorporated into the general profession. These survivals resulted from considerations, such as the distrust of specialists prior to 1875, which may or may not be pertinent at the present time. Efforts have been made, for example, to bring dentistry into the medical schools. Approaches to the same end may be observed wherever veterinary faculties cooperate with those devoted to human medicine, or where hospitals train obstetrical nurses who become as competent as good midwives.

Another aspect of training and licensing which appears in historical perspective—though not in a short-range view—is the manner in which these procedures swung from one position to another and then back again. Certain examples have been cited, as in the recent returns—or at least appeals for returns—to apprenticeship and to the licensing of second-grade personnel. More pertinent here has been cyclical behavior exhibited in the location of licensing authority. There are, in this country and in a secular age, only three possibilities. Licensing may be held in the hands of the state (as by state boards); it may be left to professional bodies; or, finally, it may be turned over to medical schools—including both "voluntary" colleges and those in state universities which operate much as do private institutions.

In the early period, between 1780 and 1830, all these possibilities were tried out in this country through state boards, medical societies and medical schools. Thereafter, until about 1875, the schools secured almost complete control of this function—often with disastrous results. Then, after the latter date, medical societies—encouraged by the better faculties—reasserted themselves and helped to reform the schools through a revival of state boards. This process, although a gradual one until 1900, proceeded rapidly during the next two decades. Yet by the 1940s schools were once more calling for independence, and some men desired a return of licensing authority to the faculties.

Such a return did not occur except in relation to specialists, and in the sense that the National Board of Medical Examiners —now so influential in this area—may be more representative of faculties than of societies at large. It seems unlikely, however, that either state boards or the voluntary National Board will advocate a revival of basic licensing by the schools.

Cyclical phenomena, of course, have not been peculiar to the medical field: they may be observed historically even within the physical sciences. But this sort of thing is naturally more common in the social sciences and in clinical medicine, which still deal with relatively inexact and often unpredictable human behavior. And in medicine these oscillations are by no means limited to education. They are just as apparent, for example, in so vital a matter as therapy.

Until about 1830, for example, "the best medicine" exhibited more or less confidence in the use of drugs; from 1830 until late in the century, increasing skepticism reached the extreme of "clinical nihilism"; then, during the present century, confidence returned and attained to new heights in the 1930s and 1940s. Yet by the 1960s, skepticism reappeared. In 1966 a conference on internal medicine heard one specialist state that 90 per cent of the antibiotics used in 19 hospitals has been wasted. What was worse, another speaker noted that more than waste was involved: as the number of drugs employed rose, so likewise did adverse reactions. Few would now deny that new drugs and procedures, used with discretion, are of great value, but it is also true that concern about iatrogenic disease is mounting. In view of all this and of other permutations, in both scientific and professional aspects of medicine, it is not surprising that licensing power has shifted from one alternative to another.

One may refer here, again, to the comparative story of the legal profession. As noted, early trends in that guild often paralleled those in medicine—reflecting the influence of a common environment. In several respects, however, legal and medical experience subsequently diverged. In the first place, admission to the bar was authorized at least until the 1870s by the courts. Law schools, unlike medical colleges, exercised no control over licensing. In this connection, law followed English rather than Continental precedents; whereas American medicine—inheriting two distinct traditions from the mother country—turned over licensing from about 1820 to 1880 to the schools rather than to medical societies. One may view law as the more fortunate profession in this connection, if it can be assumed that courts were not so tempted to admit anyone to practice as were medical faculties.

On the other hand, general reform was achieved sooner in medicine than in the legal field. Thus, A.M.A. standards for licensure (1904) appeared more than fifteen years before the American Bar Association set up guide lines for admission to practice (1921).[148] Law, moreover, was even more complicated by the existence of fifty states than was medical practice. Lawyers have been confronted by fifty somewhat different codes, whereas medicine is presumably the same in all states. It is therefore difficult to conceive of state legal reciprocity except for well-established men, or to provide national bar examinations analogous to such procedures in medicine. Law, finally, was slower than medicine in giving up the apprentice system, probably because one could just "read law" long after reading medicine and observing a preceptor ceased to be adequate in the training of physicians.

[148] See J. W. Hurst, *The Growth of American Law* (Boston: Little, Brown, 1950), pp. 276–79. On current skepticism *re* drugs, see the Philadelphia *Evening Bulletin,* April 19, 1966.

There remain, finally, rather general questions about the desirability of licensing in principle. It is doubtful if anyone, except quacks or cultists, would object today to some form of control in the medical field. Yet so thoughtful an observer as Henry Sigerist, writing in 1935, declared: "I do not believe either in tests or examinations"—a view which seems irreconcilable with licensing as we now know it. But he added that these devices were, nevertheless, a necessity in the absence of any better procedure. What Sigerist may have had in mind was the fact that test ratings cannot fully measure ability or predict subsequent achievement.[149]

This statement may seem a truism. Yet it has value as a reminder that there are always possibilities for improving the correlation of test results and final outcomes. Such progress has apparently been the experience of the National Board. Moreover, if one views licensing in a broad sense—as involving the revocation as well as the granting of rights to practice—it may be possible to improve the former as well as the latter. Dr. R. C. Derbyshire, president of the Federation of State Medical Boards, recently pointed out that more than a thousand instances of disciplinary action by state boards against physicians occurred between 1960 and 1965, and that a large percentage of these incidents involved "professional incompetence." Although the number of such cases does not seem large, and it is not clear how effective these actions were, the medical members of the boards were making some effort at professional self-discipline in the public interest.

Particularly difficult in this context are the cases of doctors who suffer from mental deterioration. That insidious process may threaten anyone but is particularly dangerous in the physician. Legal protection of patients is far from adequate. At present just twenty-three states authorize disciplinary measures

---

[149] "The History of Medical Licensure," *Jour. of the Amer. Med Assoc.*, vol. 104, (March 30, 1935), p. 1060.

concerning mental illness and fifteen of these require formal court actions. Only eight states allow their examining boards to act in such instances, and it might be more effective to transfer the control of incompetence—whatever its cause—to the boards of accredited hospitals.[150] All of which is to say that licensing procedures are still far from perfect. Yet the American profession may take some pride, in looking back over the last three centuries, in the approach toward perfection which has actually been attained.

[150] "What Should the Profession Do About the Incompetent Physician?", *Jour. of the Amer. Med. Assoc.,* vol. 194 (Dec. 20, 1965), pp. 1287–89.

Index

designer : Gerald A. Valerio
typesetter : Baltimore Type & Composition Corp.
typeface : Garamond
printer : Universal Lithographers, Inc.
paper : Perkins-Squire-GM B-10
binder : The Maple Press Company
cover material : Riverside Vellum Colonial-RV1750-Interlaken ALO-428